Nutrition for Nursing
REVIEW MODULE EDITION 8.0

Contributors

Alissa Althoff Ed.D, MSN, RN

Michelle E. Cawley, MSN, RN

Sharon M. Falk, MSN, RN, CCCTM, CHSE

Mendy Gearhart, DNP, MSN, CCCE

Lori Grace, MSN, RN

Norma Jean Henry, MSN/Ed., RN

Honey C. Holman, MSN, RN

Janean Johnson, DNP, RN, CNE

Terri Lemon, DNP, MSN, RN

Beth Cusatis Phillips, PhD,
RN, CNE, CHSE

Pamela Roland, MSN, MBA, RN

Debborah Williams, MSN, RN

Consultants

Tracey Bousquet, BSN, RN

Penny Fauber, RN, BSN, MS, PhD

INTELLECTUAL PROPERTY NOTICE

Director of content review: Kristen Lawler

Director of development: Derek Prater

Project management: Meri Ann Mason

Coordination of content review: Alissa Althoff, Honey C. Holman

Copy editing: Kelly Von Lunen, Tricia Lunt, Bethany Robertson, Kya Rodgers, Rebecca Her, Sam Shiel, Alethea Surland, Graphic World

Layout: Bethany Robertson, Maureen Bradshaw, Haylee Hedge, scottie. o

Illustrations: Randi Hardy, Graphic World

Online media: Brant Stacy, Ron Hanson, Britney Frerking, Trevor Lund

Interior book design: Spring Lenox

IMPORTANT NOTICE TO THE READER

User's Guide

Welcome to the Assessment Technologies Institute® Nutrition for Nursing Review Module Edition 8.0. The mission of ATI's Content Mastery Series® Review Modules is to provide user-friendly compendiums of nursing knowledge that will:
- Help you locate important information quickly.
- Assist in your learning efforts.
- Provide exercises for applying your nursing knowledge.
- Facilitate your entry into the nursing profession as a newly licensed nurse.

This newest edition of the Review Modules has been redesigned to optimize your learning experience. We've fit more content into less space and have done so in a way that will make it even easier for you to find and understand the information you need.

ORGANIZATION

This Review Module is organized into units covering principles of nutrition, clinical nutrition, and alterations in nutrition. Chapters within these units conform to one of two organizing principles for presenting the content.
- Nursing concepts
- Nutritional considerations for specific disorders

Nursing concepts chapters begin with an overview describing the central concept and its relevance to nursing. Subordinate themes are covered in outline form to demonstrate relationships and present the information in a clear, succinct manner.

Nutritional considerations for specific disorders chapters include an overview describing nutritional needs of clients who have the given disorder. These chapters cover assessments and data collection, nutritional guidelines, nursing interventions, and complications, if applicable.

ACTIVE LEARNING SCENARIOS AND APPLICATION EXERCISES

Each chapter includes opportunities for you to test your knowledge and to practice applying that knowledge. Active Learning Scenario exercises pose a nursing scenario and then direct you to use an ATI Active Learning Template (included at the back of this book) to record the important knowledge a nurse should apply to the scenario. An example is then provided to which you can compare your completed Active Learning Template. The Application Exercises include NCLEX-style questions, such as multiple-choice and multiple-select items, providing you with opportunities to practice answering the kinds of questions you might expect to see on ATI assessments or the NCLEX. After the Application Exercises, an answer key is provided, along with rationales.

NCLEX® CONNECTIONS

To prepare for the NCLEX, it is important to understand how the content in this Review Module is connected to the NCLEX test plan. You can find information on the detailed test plan at the National Council of State Boards of Nursing's website, www.ncsbn.org. When reviewing content in this Review Module, regularly ask yourself, "How does this content fit into the test plan, and what types of questions related to this content should I expect?"

To help you in this process, we've included NCLEX Connections at the beginning of each unit and with each question in the Application Exercises Answer Keys. The NCLEX Connections at the beginning of each unit point out areas of the detailed test plan that relate to the content within that unit. The NCLEX Connections attached to the Application Exercises Answer Keys demonstrate how each exercise fits within the detailed content outline.

These NCLEX Connections will help you understand how the detailed content outline is organized, starting with major client needs categories and subcategories and followed by related content areas and tasks. The major client needs categories are:
- Safe and Effective Care Environment
  - Management of Care
  - Safety and Infection Control
- Health Promotion and Maintenance
- Psychosocial Integrity
- Physiological Integrity
  - Basic Care and Comfort
  - Pharmacological and Parenteral Therapies
  - Reduction of Risk Potential
  - Physiological Adaptation

An NCLEX Connection might, for example, alert you that content within a unit is related to:
- Basic Care and Comfort
  - Nutrition and Oral Hydration
    - Manage the client who has an alteration in nutritional intake.

QSEN COMPETENCIES

As you use the Review Modules, you will note the integration of the Quality and Safety Education for Nurses (QSEN) competencies throughout the chapters. These competencies are integral components of the curriculum of many nursing programs in the United States and prepare you to provide safe, high-quality care as a newly licensed nurse. Icons appear to draw your attention to the six QSEN competencies.

Safety: The minimization of risk factors that could cause injury or harm while promoting quality care and maintaining a secure environment for clients, self, and others.

Patient-Centered Care: The provision of caring and compassionate, culturally sensitive care that addresses clients' physiological, psychological, sociological, spiritual, and cultural needs, preferences, and values.

Evidence-Based Practice: The use of current knowledge from research and other credible sources, on which to base clinical judgment and client care.

Informatics: The use of information technology as a communication and information-gathering tool that supports clinical decision-making and scientifically based nursing practice.

Quality Improvement: Care related and organizational processes that involve the development and implementation of a plan to improve health care services and better meet clients' needs.

Teamwork and Collaboration: The delivery of client care in partnership with multidisciplinary members of the health care team to achieve continuity of care and positive client outcomes.

ICONS

Icons are used throughout the Review Modules to draw your attention to particular areas. Keep an eye out for these icons.

N This icon is used for NCLEX Connections.

G This icon indicates gerontological considerations, or knowledge specific to the care of older adult clients.

Qs This icon is used for content related to safety and is a QSEN competency. When you see this icon, take note of safety concerns or steps that nurses can take to ensure client safety and a safe environment.

QPCC This icon is a QSEN competency that indicates the importance of a holistic approach to providing care.

QEBP This icon, a QSEN competency, points out the integration of research into clinical practice.

QI This icon is a QSEN competency and highlights the use of information technology to support nursing practice.

QQI This icon is used to focus on the QSEN competency of integrating planning processes to meet clients' needs.

QTC This icon highlights the QSEN competency of care delivery using an interprofessional approach.

QSDoH This icon highlights content related to social determinants of health.

M◇ This icon appears at the top-right of pages and indicates availability of an online media supplement, such as a graphic, animation, or video. If you have an electronic copy of the Review Module, this icon will appear alongside clickable links to media supplements. If you have a hard copy version of the Review Module, visit www.atitesting.com for details on how to access these features.

FEEDBACK

ATI welcomes feedback regarding this Review Module. Please provide comments to comments@atitesting.com.

As needed updates to the Review Modules are identified, changes to the text are made for subsequent printings of the book and for subsequent releases of the electronic version. For the printed books, print runs are based on when existing stock is depleted. For the electronic versions, a number of factors influence the update schedule. As such, ATI encourages faculty and students to refer to the Review Module addendums for information on what updates have been made. These addendums—which are available in the Help/FAQs on the student site and the Resources/eBooks & Active Learning on the faculty site—are updated regularly and always include the most current information on updates to the Review Modules.

Table of Contents

UNIT 2 · *Clinical Nutrition*

UNIT 3 · *Alterations in Nutrition*

References · 99

Active Learning Templates · A1

When reviewing the following chapters, keep in mind the relevant topics and tasks of the NCLEX outline:

Health Promotion and Maintenance

AGING PROCESS
Provide care and education for the newborn, infant, and toddler client from birth through 2 years of age.

Provide care and education for the adult client ages 65 years and over.

ANTE-/INTRA-/POSTPARTUM AND NEWBORN CARE: Provide prenatal care and education.

HEALTH PROMOTION/DISEASE PREVENTION: Educate the client on actions to promote/maintain health and prevent disease.

HEALTH SCREENING: Perform targeted screening assessments.

Basic Care and Comfort

NUTRITION AND ORAL HYDRATION
Consider client choices regarding meeting nutritional requirements and/or maintaining dietary restrictions, including mention of specific food items.

Initiate calorie counts for clients.

Apply knowledge of mathematics to client nutrition.

Physiological Adaptation

FLUID AND ELECTROLYTE IMBALANCES: Manage the care of the client who has a fluid and electrolyte imbalance.

UNIT 1 PRINCIPLES OF NUTRITION

CHAPTER 1 *Sources of Nutrition*

Nutrients absorbed in the diet determine, to a large degree, the health of the body. Deficiencies or excesses can contribute to a poor state of health. Essential nutrients are those that the body cannot manufacture, and the absence of essential nutrients can cause deficiency diseases.

Components of nutritive sources are carbohydrates and fiber, protein, lipids (fats), vitamins, minerals and electrolytes, and water. Carbohydrates, fats, and proteins are all energy-yielding nutrients. A healthy eating pattern includes foods that provide all essential nutrients and allows a broad assortment of food sources.

DIETARY REFERENCE INTAKES

Dietary Reference Intakes (DRIs) are developed by the Institute of Medicine's Standing Committee on the Scientific Evaluation of Dietary Reference Intakes.

- DRIs are useful in understanding the food intake patterns of large groups, planning nutrition program standards (Supplemental Nutrition Assistance program [SNAP]), and helping individuals.
- DRIs are comprised of the following reference values.
  - Recommended Dietary Allowances (RDAs): The amount of a particular nutrient that most healthy people with a similar life-stage and sex will need to decrease the risk of chronic disease
  - Estimated Average Requirement (EAR): The amount of a nutrient required to meet basic requirements for half of the people in a particular population. This reference is often used by researchers and policy makers and is used to help determine RDAs.
  - Adequate Intake (AI): The amount of a nutrient that most people in a group or population consume. This is helpful when there is not enough data to establish an RDA for a nutrient.
  - Tolerable Upper Intake Level (UL): The upper limit on the amount of a particular nutrient or the maximum an individual should consume. ULs are used when a nutrient is known to have adverse effects.
  - Acceptable Macronutrient Distribution Ranges (AMDRs): The recommended percentages of intake for energy-yielding nutrients (carbohydrates, fat, protein).
- Clients can use DRIs as a guide for nutrition intake but should also consider individual factors that increase nutrient needs (disease, injury).

Carbohydrates and fiber

All carbohydrates are organic compounds composed of carbon, hydrogen, and oxygen (CHO). The main function of carbohydrates is to provide energy for the body.

- The average minimum amount (DRI) of carbohydrates needed to fuel the brain is 130 g/day for adults and children. Median carbohydrate intake is 305 g/day for males aged 20 years and older, and 228 g/day for adults, children, and females in the same age range. The AMDR for carbohydrates is 45% to 65% of calories.
- Carbohydrates provide energy for cellular work and help to regulate protein and fat metabolism. Adequate amounts of protein in the diet creates a protein-sparing effect, which results in protein being spared from energy use to perform its other essential functions. Brain and nervous system tissue require carbohydrates for maximum effective functioning.

TYPES OF CARBOHYDRATES

Carbohydrates are classified according to the number of saccharide units making up their structure.

Monosaccharides: simple carbohydrates (glucose, fructose, and galactose)

Disaccharides: simple carbohydrates (sucrose, lactose, and maltose)

Polysaccharides: complex carbohydrates (starch, fiber, and glycogen)

CONSIDERATIONS

- The liver converts fructose and galactose into glucose, which is then released into the bloodstream. This elevates blood glucose levels, which causes the release of insulin from the pancreas. With insulin production, glucose is moved out of the bloodstream into cells in order to meet energy needs.
- The body digests 95% of starch within 1 to 4 hr after ingestion. Digestion occurs mainly in the small intestine using pancreatic amylase to reduce complex carbohydrates into disaccharides.
- Glycogen is the stored carbohydrate energy source found in the liver and muscles. It is a vital source of backup energy but is only available in limited supply.
- To maintain glucose levels between meals, glucose is released through the breakdown of liver glycogen.
- Digestible carbohydrates provide 4 cal/g of energy and make blood glucose levels more stable.

1.1 Carbohydrates at a glance

	EXAMPLE (SOURCES)	FUNCTION
Monosaccharides	Glucose (corn syrup), fructose (fruits), galactose (found in milk)	Basic energy for cells
Disaccharides	Sucrose (table sugar), lactose (milk sugar), maltose (malt sugar)	Energy, aids calcium and phosphorus absorption (lactose)
Polysaccharides	Starches (grains, legumes, root vegetables), fiber (whole grains, fruits, vegetables)	Energy storage (starches), digestive aid (fiber)

Fiber

Fiber is categorized as a carbohydrate.
- Dietary fiber is the substance in plant foods that is indigestible. Types are pectin, gum, cellulose, and oligosaccharides.
- Fiber is important for proper bowel elimination. It adds bulk to the feces and stimulates peristalsis to ease elimination.
- Fiber helps to lower cholesterol and lessen the incidence of intestinal cancers. It has also been shown to help keep blood glucose levels stable by slowing the rate of glucose absorption.
- Total fiber AI is 25 g/day for females and 38 g/day for males.
- The fermentation and metabolization of fiber in the colon provide 1.5 to 2.5 cal/g of energy, depending on the type.

Proteins

Proteins are provided by plant and animal sources. They are formed by linking amino acids in various combinations for specific use by the body.

TYPES OF PROTEINS

There are two types of proteins. Each is obtained from the diet in various ways.

Complete proteins, from animal sources and soy, contain sufficient amounts of all nine essential amino acids.

Incomplete proteins, generally from plant sources, can contain an insufficient number or quantity of amino acids, which limits the ability for protein synthesis.
- **Complementary proteins** are incomplete proteins that, when combined, provide a complete protein. It is not necessary to consume complementary proteins at the same time to form a complete protein; instead, consuming a variety of complementary proteins over the course of the day is sufficient.
- Examples of incomplete protein pairs that provide complete protein include black beans with rice and hummus with crackers.

CONSIDERATIONS

- Proteins have many metabolic functions.
  - Tissue-building and maintenance
  - Balance of nitrogen and water
  - Backup energy
  - Support of metabolic processes
    - Nitrogen balance
    - Transportation of nutrients, other vital substances
  - Support of the immune system
  - Facilitating acid-base, fluid, and electrolyte balance
  - Formation of neurotransmitters, enzymes antibodies, peptide hormones, breast milk, mucus, histamine, and sperm

- Three main factors influence the body's requirement for protein.
  - Tissue growth needs
  - Quality of the dietary protein
  - Added needs due to illness
- The RDA of protein is 0.8 g/kg for healthy adults. Protein's acceptable macronutrient distribution range (AMDR) for adults is 10% to 35% of total calories.
- Underconsumption can lead to protein energy malnutrition (PEM). Kwashiorkor and marasmus are two disorders caused by extreme PEM. These serious disorders are caused by a lack of protein ingestion.
- Protein provides 4 cal/g of energy.

Lipids

- The chemical group of fats is called lipids, and they are available from many sources.
  - Dark meat
  - Poultry skin
  - Dairy foods
  - Added oils (margarine, butter, shortening, oils, lard)
- Fat is an essential nutrient for the body. It serves as a concentrated form of stored energy for the body and supplies important tissue needs.
  - Hormone production
  - Structural material for cell walls
  - Protective padding for vital organs
  - Insulation to maintain body temperature
  - Covering for nerve fibers
  - Aid in the absorption of fat-soluble vitamins

TYPES OF FATS

Fats are divided into three categories: triglycerides, phospholipids, and sterols. Triglycerides are further comprised of fatty acids, which include saturated fatty acids and unsaturated fatty acids.

Triglycerides

Triglycerides total 95% of fat in food. They combine with glycerol to supply energy to the body, allow fat-soluble vitamin transport, and form adipose tissue that protects internal organs.

Saturated fatty acids are solid at room temperature and are found primarily in animal sources.

Unsaturated fatty acids, including monounsaturated and polyunsaturated fatty acids, are usually from plant sources and help reduce health risks.
- Sources of monounsaturated fatty acids include olives, canola oil, avocado, peanuts, and other nuts.
- Sources of polyunsaturated fatty acids include corn, wheat germ, soybean, safflower, sunflower, and fish.

Essential fatty acids, made from broken down fats, must be supplied by the diet. Essential fatty acids, including omega-3 and omega-6, are used to support blood clotting, blood pressure, inflammatory responses, and many other metabolic processes.

Phospholipids

Phospholipids (e.g., lecithin) are important to cell membrane structure, as well as the transport of fat-soluble substances across the cell membrane.

Sterols

Sterols (e.g., cholesterol) are found in the tissues of animals, and are not an essential nutrient because the liver is able to produce enough to meet needs.

If cholesterol is consumed in excess, it can build up in the tissues, causing congestion and increasing the risk for cardiovascular disease.

CONSIDERATIONS

- The AMDR for fats is approximately 20% to 35% of total calories. 10% or less of total calories should come from saturated fat sources.
- A low intake of dietary cholesterol is associated with reduced risks of cardiovascular disease (CVD) and obesity.
- A diet high in fat is linked to CVD, hypertension, and diabetes mellitus.
  - The exception is for children under 2 years of age, who need a higher amount of fat to form brain tissue.
  - Conversely, a diet with less than 10% of fat cannot supply adequate amounts of essential fatty acids and results in a cachectic (wasting) state.
- The majority of lipid metabolism occurs after fat reaches the small intestine, where the gallbladder secretes concentrated bile, which acts as an emulsifier and enables the breakdown of fat down into smaller particles for digestion. At the same time, the pancreas secretes pancreatic lipase, which breaks down fat. Intestinal cells absorb the majority of the end products of digestion, with some being excreted in the feces.
  - **Very-low-density lipoproteins (VLDL)** carry triglycerides to the cells.
  - **Low-density lipoproteins (LDL)** carry cholesterol to the tissue cells.
  - **High-density lipoproteins (HDL)** remove excess cholesterol from the cells and transport it to the liver for disposal.
- Lipids provide 9 cal/g of energy and are the densest form of stored energy.

Vitamins

Vitamins are organic substances required for many enzymatic reactions. The main function of vitamins is to be a catalyst for metabolic functions and chemical reactions.
- There are 13 essential vitamins, each having a specialized function.
- There are two classes of vitamins.
  - **Water-soluble:** Vitamins C and B-complex
  - **Fat-soluble:** Vitamins A, D, E, and K
- Vitamins yield no usable energy for the body, but they are needed for energy to be metabolized.

WATER-SOLUBLE VITAMINS

Vitamin C

Vitamin C (ascorbic acid) aids in tissue building and metabolic reactions (healing, collagen formation, iron absorption, immune system function).
- Vitamin C is found in citrus fruits (oranges, lemons), tomatoes, peppers, green leafy vegetables, and strawberries.
- Stress and illness, as well as cigarette smoking, increase the need for vitamin C. Cigarette smokers are advised to increase vitamin C intake by 35 mg/day due to increased oxidative stress and metabolic turnover.
- Severe deficiency causes scurvy, a hemorrhagic disease with diffuse tissue bleeding, painful limbs/joints, weak bones, and swollen gums/loose teeth. While scurvy can be fatal, it can also be cured with moderate doses of vitamin C for several days.

B-complex vitamins

B-complex vitamins have many functions in cell metabolism. Each one has a varied duty. Many partner with other B vitamins for metabolic reactions. Most affect energy, metabolism, and neurologic function. Sources for B vitamins almost always include green leafy vegetables and unprocessed or enriched grains.

Thiamin (B_1) functions as a coenzyme in energy metabolism, promotes appetite, and assists with muscle actions through its role in nerve functioning.
- Deficiency results in beriberi (ataxia, confusion, anorexia, tachycardia), headache, weight loss, and fatigue.
- Food sources are widespread in almost all plant and animal tissues, especially meats, grains, and legumes.

Riboflavin (B_2) works as a coenzyme to release energy from cells.
- Deficiency results in cheilosis (manifestations include scales and cracks on lips and in corners of the mouth), smooth/swollen red tongue (also called glossitis), and dermatitis of the ears, nose, and mouth.
- Dietary sources include milk, meats, and dark leafy vegetables.

Niacin (B_3) aids in the metabolism of fats, glucose, and alcohol, and synthesis of steroid hormones, cholesterol, and fatty acids.
- Deficiency causes pellagra (manifestations include sun-sensitive skin lesions, and gastrointestinal issues with impaired food digestion and excretion, as well as nutrient absorption and neurologic findings [anxiety, insomnia, confusion, paranoia]).
- Sources include meats, legumes, milk, whole grain and enriched breads and cereals.

Pyridoxine/Vitamin (B_6) is needed for cellular function and synthesis of hemoglobin, neurotransmitters, and niacin.
- Deficiency causes macrocytic anemia and CNS disturbances.
- High intake of supplements can cause sensory neuropathy.
- Widespread food sources include meats, grains, and legumes.

Pantothenic acid is involved in the metabolism of carbohydrates, fats, and proteins as part of coenzyme A.
- Deficiency is extremely rare but results in generalized body system failure.
- Rich sources include meats, whole grain cereals, dried peas, and beans.

Biotin serves as a coenzyme used in fatty acid synthesis, amino acid metabolism, and the formation of glucose.
- Deficiency is rare but results in neurologic findings (depression, fatigue), hair loss, and scaly red rash.
- Widespread food sources include eggs, milk, and dark green vegetables.

Folate is required for hemoglobin and amino acid synthesis, new cell synthesis, and prevention of neural tube defects in utero. (Folic acid is the synthetic form.)
- Deficiency causes megaloblastic anemia, CNS disturbances, and fetal neural tube defects (spina bifida, anencephaly). It is important that all clients of child-bearing age get an adequate amount of folate due to neural tube formation occurring early in gestation, often before a client knows they are pregnant. Q EBP
- Folate occurs naturally in a variety of foods including liver, dark-green leafy vegetables, orange juice, and legumes.

Cobalamin (B₁₂) is necessary for folate activation and red blood cell maturation.
- Deficiency causes pernicious anemia and is seen mostly in clients who follow a strict vegan diet (B12 is found solely in foods of animal origin) and those who have an absence of intrinsic factor needed for absorption of B12.
- Sources include meat, shellfish, eggs, and dairy products.

FAT-SOLUBLE VITAMINS

- All fat-soluble vitamins have the possibility for toxicity due to their ability to be stored in the body for long periods of time.
- Absorption of fat-soluble vitamins is dependent on the body's ability to absorb dietary fat. Fat digestion can be interrupted by any number of conditions, particularly those that affect the secretion of fat-converting enzymes, and conditions of the small intestine. Clients who have cystic fibrosis, celiac disease, Crohn's disease, or intestinal bypasses are at risk for deficiencies.
- Clients who have liver disease should be careful not to take more than the daily recommendations of fat-soluble vitamins, as excess is stored in the liver and adipose tissue.

Vitamin A

Vitamin A (retinol, beta-carotene) contributes to vision health, tissue strength and growth, and embryonic development. Retinoids are found in animal foods and are the active form of vitamin A. Carotenoids are found in plants and are a precursor form of vitamin A, which the body converts to the usable form as needed.
- Care should be taken when administered to clients who are pregnant as some forms have teratogenic effects on the fetus.
- Deficiency results in vision changes, xerophthalmia (dryness and hardening of the cornea), GI disturbances, and hyperkeratosis.
- Food sources include fatty fish, egg yolks, butter, cream, and dark yellow/orange fruits and vegetables (carrots, yams, apricots, squash, cantaloupe).
- Toxicity can result from retinoids and is more common in clients who are taking vitamin A supplements.

1.2 Water-soluble vitamins at a glance

	MAJOR ACTIONS	MAJOR SOURCES	DEFICIENCY
Vitamin C (ascorbic acid)	Antioxidant, tissue building, iron absorption	Citrus fruits and juices, vegetables	Scurvy, decreased iron absorption, bleeding gums
Thiamin (B₁)	Muscle energy, energy metabolism	Meats, grains, legumes	Beriberi, headache, weight loss, fatigue
Riboflavin (B₂)	Assists with releasing energy from cells	Milk, meats, dark leafy vegetables	Skin eruptions, cracked lips, red swollen tongue
Niacin (B₃)	Metabolism of fat, glucose, and alcohol; synthesis of fatty acids, cholesterol, and steroid hormones	Liver, nuts, legumes	Pellagra, skin lesions, GI and CNS findings, dementia
Pantothenic acid	Carbohydrate, fat, and protein metabolism	Meats, whole grain cereals, dried peas and beans.	Rare / Generalized body system failure
Pyridoxine (B₆)	Cellular function, heme and neurotransmitter synthesis	Meats, grains, and legumes	Macrocytic anemia, CNS disturbances, poor growth
Folate	Synthesis of amino acids and hemoglobin, formation of fetal neural tube	Liver, green leafy vegetables, legumes	Megaloblastic anemia, CNS disturbance
Cobalamin (B₁₂)	Folate activation, red blood cell maturation	Meats, clams, oysters, eggs, dairy products	Pernicious anemia, GI findings, poor muscle coordination, paresthesia of the hands and feet
Biotin	Fatty acid synthesis, amino acid metabolism, glucose formation	Eggs, milk, dark green vegetables	Rare; scaly rash, hair loss, depression, fatigue

Vitamin D

Vitamin D assists in the absorption of calcium and phosphorus and aids in bone mineralization.
- Sunlight enables the body to synthesize vitamin D in the skin.
- Deficiency results in bone demineralization, and extreme deficiency can cause rickets and osteomalacia. Excess consumption can cause hypercalcemia.
- Food sources include fatty fish, eggs, and fortified products (ready-to-eat cereals, milk, orange juice).

VITAMIN E

Vitamin E is an antioxidant that helps to preserve lung and red blood cell membranes.
- Deficiency rare but results in anemia and can cause edema and skin lesions in infants.
- Food sources include vegetable oils and certain nuts.

VITAMIN K

Vitamin K assists in blood clotting and bone maintenance.
- Deficiency results in increased bleeding time.
- Used as an antidote for excess anticoagulants (warfarin).
- Vitamin K is found in carrots, eggs, and dark green vegetables (spinach, broccoli, asparagus).

Minerals and electrolytes

Minerals are inorganic elements, available in an abundance of food sources, and used at every cellular level for metabolic exchanges. Minerals are divided into major and trace.

Electrolytes are electrically charged minerals that cause physiological reactions that maintain homeostasis. Major electrolytes include sodium, potassium, and chloride.

MAJOR MINERALS

Major minerals occur in larger amounts (more than 5 g) in the body, and 100 mg or more is required through dietary sources each day. The seven major minerals are calcium, phosphorus, sodium, potassium, magnesium, chloride, and sulfur.

Sodium (Na)

MAJOR ACTIONS: Maintains fluid volume, allows muscle contractions, contributes to nerve impulses

MAJOR SOURCES: Table salt, added salts, processed foods

FINDINGS OF DEFICIENCY: Muscle cramping, memory loss, anorexia

FINDINGS OF EXCESS: Fluid retention, hypertension, disorientation

NURSING ACTIONS: Monitor level of consciousness, edema, and blood pressure.

Potassium (K)

MAJOR ACTIONS: Maintains fluid volume inside cells, muscle action

MAJOR SOURCES: Oranges, dried fruits, tomatoes, avocados, dried peas, meats, broccoli, bananas, dairy products, meats, whole grains, potatoes

FINDINGS OF DEFICIENCY: Dysrhythmias, muscle cramps, confusion

FINDINGS OF EXCESS: Dysrhythmia, muscle weakness, irritability, confusion, numbness in extremities

NURSING ACTIONS: Monitor cardiac status and ECG. Give oral preparations (tabs, elixirs) with meals to minimize GI irritation.

Chloride (Cl)

MAJOR ACTIONS: Assists with intracellular and extracellular fluid balance and aids acid-based balance and digestion

MAJOR SOURCES: Table salt, added salts, processed foods

FINDINGS OF DEFICIENCY: Rare; muscle cramps, anorexia

FINDINGS OF EXCESS: Vomiting

NURSING ACTIONS: Monitor sodium levels.

1.3 Fat-soluble vitamins at a glance

	MAJOR ACTIONS	MAJOR SOURCES	DEFICIENCY
Vitamin A	Normal vision, tissue strength, growth and immune system function	Orange/yellow fruits and vegetables, fatty fish, dairy	Reduced night vision, dry/thick corneas, mucosa changes
Vitamin D	Maintain blood calcium and phosphorus, aid in bone development	Fish, fortified dairy products, egg yolks, sunlight	Low blood calcium, fragile bones, rickets, osteomalacia in adults
Vitamin E	Protects vitamin A from oxidation	Vegetable oils, grains, nuts, dark green vegetables	Anemia, edema and skin lesions in infants
Vitamin K	Essential for prothrombin synthesis, aids in bone metabolism	Green leafy vegetables, eggs	Increased bleeding times

Calcium (Ca)

MAJOR ACTIONS: Bones/teeth formation, blood pressure, blood clotting, nerve transmission

MAJOR SOURCES: Dairy, broccoli, kale, fortified grains

FINDINGS OF DEFICIENCY: Tetany, positive Chvostek's and Trousseau's signs, ECG changes, osteoporosis in adults, poor growth in children

FINDINGS OF EXCESS: Constipation, renal stones, lethargy, depressed deep-tendon reflexes

NURSING ACTIONS: Monitor ECG and respiratory status. Give PO tabs with vitamin D.

Magnesium (Mg)

MAJOR ACTIONS: Bone formation, catalyst for many enzyme reactions, nerve/muscle function, smooth muscle relaxation

MAJOR SOURCES: Green leafy vegetables, nuts, whole grains, tuna, halibut, chocolate

FINDINGS OF DEFICIENCY: Weakness, dysrhythmias, convulsions, increased blood pressure, anorexia

FINDINGS OF EXCESS: Diarrhea, nausea, muscle weakness, hypotension, bradycardia, lethargy

NURSING ACTIONS: Follow seizure precautions, and monitor level of consciousness and vital signs. Qs

Phosphorus (P)

MAJOR ACTIONS: Energy transfer of RNA/DNA, acid-base balance, bone and teeth formation

MAJOR SOURCES: Dairy, peas, meat, eggs, legumes

FINDINGS OF DEFICIENCY: Unknown

FINDINGS OF EXCESS: Decreased blood calcium levels

NURSING ACTIONS: Evaluate the use of antacids (note type) and the use of alcohol (alcohol impairs absorption).

Sulfur (S)

MAJOR ACTIONS: A component of vitamin structure, by-product of protein metabolism

MAJOR SOURCES: Proteins

FINDINGS OF DEFICIENCY: Only seen in severe protein malnourishment

FINDINGS OF EXCESS: Toxicity does not result in any health issues

NURSING ACTIONS: Sulfur levels are not usually monitored.

TRACE MINERALS

Trace minerals, also called micronutrients, are required by the body in amounts of less than 5 g, and 20 mg or less is required through dietary sources each day. The nine trace elements are iron, iodine, zinc, copper, manganese, chromium, selenium, molybdenum, and fluoride.

Iodine

Iodine is used for synthesis of thyroxine, the thyroid hormone that helps regulate metabolism. Iodine is taken up by the thyroid. When iodine is lacking, the thyroid gland enlarges, creating a goiter. Too much iodine can result in thyrotoxicosis.
- Grown food sources vary widely and are dependent on the iodine content of the soil in which they were grown.
- Seafood provides a good amount of iodine. Table salt in the U.S. is fortified with iodine, so deficiencies are not as prevalent.
- The RDA is 150 mcg for adults.

Iron

Iron is responsible for oxygen distribution to hemoglobin and myoglobin.
- The body recycles unused iron from dying red blood cells and stores it for later use.
- Iron in food consists of two forms: heme iron found in meat, fish, and poultry and non-heme iron found in grains, legumes, and vegetables.
- Iron supplements can cause constipation, nausea, vomiting, diarrhea, and teeth discoloration (liquid form). They can be taken with food to avert gastrointestinal manifestations, and nurses should encourage fresh fruits, vegetables, and a high-fiber diet.
- Supplements that are unneeded can become toxic.
- Vitamin C increases the absorption of iron.
- Clients during the menstruating years, older infants and toddlers, and pregnant clients are at risk for iron deficiency anemia.
- Toxicity can occur when there is too much iron stored in the body.

Fluoride

Fluoride forms a bond with calcium and thus accumulates in calcified body tissue (bones and teeth). Water with added fluoride protects against dental cavities.
- Deficiency can result in dental caries and increase the risk for osteoporosis.
- Toxicity can result in fluorosis, itching, and chest pain.

Water

Water is the most basic of nutrients. The body can maintain itself for several weeks on its food stores of energy, but it cannot survive without water/hydration for more than a few days. Water makes up the largest portion of our total body weight and is crucial for all fluid and cellular functions.
- Fluid balance is essential for optimum health and bodily function.
- The balance of fluid is a dynamic process regulated by the release of hormones.
- Water leaves the body via the kidneys, skin, lungs, and feces. The greatest elimination is through the kidneys. Other loss factors include bleeding, vomiting, and rapid respirations.

- To maintain a balance between intake and output, intake should approximate output. Healthy adults lose approximately 1000 mL of water daily through insensible losses (respirations, skin, fecal), and to get rid of metabolic wastes needs to excrete at least 500 mL of urine daily. Therefore, the minimum daily amount of water intake needed is 1,500 mL.
- Most water intake is from drinking fluids; water is also present in solid sources (lettuce, gelatin, soup, melons). Under normal conditions, the AI for adult water intake for females is 2.7 L/day, of which 2.2 L should be from fluids; and for males 3.7 L/day, of which 3 L should be from fluids. ⓠEBP
- Additional hydration can be required for athletes, persons with fever/illness (vomiting, diarrhea), and those in hot climate conditions. Fluid replacement can occur orally, enterally, or IV.
- Young children and older adults dehydrate more rapidly.
- Assessment for proper hydration should include skin turgor, mental status, orthostatic blood pressures, urine output and concentration, and moistness of mucous membranes.
- Thirst is a late indicator of the need for hydration, especially in older adults. ⓖ
- Some individuals can have an aversion to drinking water and should be encouraged to explore other options (fresh fruits, fruit juices, flavored gelatin, frozen treats, soups).
- Caffeinated drinks have a mild diuretic effect. However, tolerance develops in clients who regularly consume caffeinated beverages, which results in little to no effect on fluid volume.

Phytonutrients

Also called phytochemicals, phytonutrients occur naturally in plants. They can have positive health effects (detoxifying the body, stimulating the immune system, promoting hormone balance, serving as antioxidants).
- They are found in fruits, vegetables, green tea, legumes, whole grains, and broccoli.
- No recommendations for intake of phytonutrients exist at this time.

Vitamin D

Fatty fish, eggs, and fortified products (ready-to-eat cereals, milk, orange juice)

Calcium

Dairy, broccoli, kale, fortified grains

Sodium

Table salt, added salts, processed foods

Potassium

Oranges, dried fruits, tomatoes, avocados, dried peas, meats, broccoli, bananas, dairy products, meats, whole grains, potato

Vitamin A

Fatty fish, egg yolks, butter, cream, and dark yellow/orange fruits and vegetables (carrots, yams, apricots, squash, cantaloupe)

Vitamin E

Vegetable oils and certain nuts

Application Exercises

1. A nurse is discussing health problems associated with nutrient deficiencies with a group of clients. Which of the following conditions is associated with a deficiency of vitamin C? (Select all that apply.)
   A. Dysrhythmias
   B. Scurvy
   C. Pernicious anemia
   D. Megaloblastic anemia
   E. Bleeding gums

2. A nurse is conducting a nutritional class on minerals and electrolytes. The nurse should include which of the following foods as a major source of magnesium?
   A. Tuna
   B. Tomatoes
   C. Eggs
   D. Oranges

3. A nurse is reviewing information about dietary intake of iron with a client who has anemia. Which of the following is a non-heme source of iron?
   A. Ground beef
   B. Dried beans
   C. Salmon
   D. Turkey

4. A nurse is reviewing dietary recommendations with a group of clients at a health fair. Which of the following information should the nurse include?
   A. "Fats should be 5% to 15% of daily calorie intake."
   B. "Make protein 10% to 35% of total calories each day."
   C. "Consume 1,500 mL of water from liquids and solids daily."
   D. "The body needs 40 mg of iron each day."

Application Exercises Key

1. B, E. **CORRECT:** When taking actions, the nurse should inform the clients that scurvy and bleeding gums are health conditions associated with a vitamin C deficiency.

   Ⓝ *NCLEX® Connection: Physiological Adaptation, Illness Management*

2. A. **CORRECT:** When taking actions, the nurse should include the information that tuna and halibut are major sources of magnesium.

   Ⓝ *NCLEX® Connection: Physiological Adaptation, Fluid and Electrolyte Imbalances*

3. B. **CORRECT:** When taking actions, the nurse should review with the client that dried beans provide non-heme iron, as do other legumes, vegetables, and grains.

   Ⓝ *NCLEX® Connection: Basic Care and Comfort, Nutrition and Oral Hydration*

4. B. **CORRECT:** When taking actions, the nurse should include in their review that the dietary recommendation for protein intake is 10% to 35% of total daily calories.

   Ⓝ *NCLEX® Connection: Basic Care and Comfort, Nutrition and Oral Hydration*

Active Learning Scenario

A school nurse is conducting a nutritional class for a group of athletes. Use the ATI Active Learning Template: Basic Concept to complete this item.

RELATED CONTENT

- Describe two types of protein.
- Describe complimentary proteins.
- Describe three main factors influencing the body's requirement for protein.

Active Learning Scenario Key

Using the ATI Active Learning Template: Basic Concept

RELATED CONTENT

- Types of protein
  - Complete proteins, from animal sources and soy, contain sufficient amounts of all nine essential amino acids.
  - Incomplete proteins, generally from plant sources, can contain an insufficient number or quantity of amino acids, which limits the ability for protein synthesis.
- Complementary proteins
  - Complementary proteins are those food sources that are incomplete proteins eaten alone, but together are equivalent to a complete protein. It is not necessary to consume complementary proteins at the same time to form a complete protein; instead, consuming a variety of complementary proteins over the course of the day is sufficient.
- Main factors influencing the body's requirement for protein
  - Tissue growth needs
  - Quality of the dietary protein
  - Added needs due to illness

Ⓝ *NCLEX® Connection: Health Promotion and Maintenance, Health Promotion/Disease Prevention*

UNIT 1   PRINCIPLES OF NUTRITION

CHAPTER 2   *Ingestion, Digestion, Absorption, and Metabolism*

Ingestion is the process of consuming food by the mouth and moving it through the digestive system. Digestion is a systemic process that includes the breakdown and absorption of nutrients.

Absorption occurs as components of nutrients pass through the digestive system into the bloodstream and lymphatic system.

Metabolism is the sum of all chemical processes that occur on a cellular level to maintain homeostasis. Metabolism is comprised of catabolism (the breaking down of substances with the resultant release of energy) and anabolism (the use of energy to build or repair substances).

Energy nutrients are metabolized to provide carbon dioxide, water, and adenosine triphosphate (ATP). Excess energy nutrients are stored; glucose is converted to glycogen and stored in the liver and muscle tissue; surplus glucose is converted to fat; glycerol and fatty acids are reassembled into triglycerides and stored in adipose tissue; and amino acids make body proteins. The liver removes nitrogen from amino acids, and the remaining product is converted to glucose or fat for energy. Body cells first use available ATP for growth and repair, then use glycogen and stored fat.

METABOLIC RATE

Metabolic rate refers to the speed at which food energy is burned.

- **Basal metabolic rate (BMR)**, also called basal energy expenditure (BEE), refers to the amount of energy used in 24 hr for involuntary activities of the body (maintaining body temperature, heartbeat, circulation, and respirations). This rate is determined while at rest and following a 12-hr fast.
- **Resting metabolic rate (RMR)**, also called resting energy expenditure (REE), refers to the calories needed for involuntary activities of the body at rest. This rate does not consider the 12-hr fast criteria.
- BMR is affected by lean body mass and hormones. Body surface area, age, and sex are also factors that contribute to BMR.
- In general, individuals who are assigned male sex at birth have a higher metabolic rate than individuals who are assigned female sex at birth due to their higher amount of body muscle and decreased amount of fat.
- Thyroid function tests can be used as an indirect measure of BMR.
- Acute stress causes an increase in metabolism, blood glucose levels, and protein catabolism.
  - A major nutritional concern during acute stress is protein deficiency as stress hormones break down protein at a very rapid rate.
  - Protein deficiency increases the risk of complications from severe trauma or critical illness (skin breakdown, delayed wound healing, infections, organ failure, ulcers, impaired medication tolerance).
  - Protein requirements can be increased to more than 2 g/kg of body weight, or up to 25% of total calories, depending on the client's age and prior nutritional status. Q EBP
- Any catabolic illness (surgery, extensive burns) increases the body's requirement for calories to meet the demands of an increased BMR.
- Disease and sepsis also increase metabolic demands and can lead to starvation/death.

FACTORS AFFECTING METABOLIC RATE

INCREASE BMR
- Lean, muscular body build
- Exposure to extreme temperatures
- Prolonged stress
- Rapid growth periods (infancy, puberty)
- Pregnancy and lactation
- Physical conditioning

DECREASE BMR
- Short, overweight body build
- Starvation/malnutrition
- Age-related loss of lean body masses Ⓖ

CONDITIONS

INCREASE METABOLISM
- Fever
- Involuntary muscle tremors (shivering, Parkinson's)
- Hyperthyroidism
- Cancer
- Cardiac failure
- Burns
- Surgery/wound healing
- HIV/AIDS

DECREASE METABOLISM: Hypothyroidism

Medications

INCREASE BMR
- Epinephrine
- Levothyroxine
- Ephedrine sulfate

DECREASE BMR
- Opioids
- Muscle relaxants
- Barbiturates

NITROGEN BALANCE

Nitrogen balance refers to the difference between the daily intake and excretion of nitrogen. It is also an indicator of tissue integrity. A healthy adult experiencing a stable weight is in nitrogen equilibrium, also known as neutral nitrogen balance.

Positive nitrogen balance indicates that the intake of nitrogen exceeds excretion. Specifically, the body builds more tissue than it breaks down. This normally occurs during periods of growth: infancy, childhood, adolescence, pregnancy, and lactation.

Negative nitrogen balance indicates that the excretion of nitrogen exceeds intake. The individual is receiving insufficient protein, and the body is breaking down more tissue than it is building, as seen during periods of illness, trauma, aging, and malnutrition.

ASSESSMENT/DATA COLLECTION

- Weight and history of recent weight patterns
- Medical history for diseases that affect metabolism and nitrogen balance
- Extent of traumatic injuries, as appropriate
- Fluid and electrolyte status
- Laboratory values: albumin, transferrin, glucose, creatinine
- Clinical findings of malnutrition: pitting edema, hair loss, wasted appearance
- Medication adverse effects that can affect nutrition
- Usual 24-hr dietary intake
- Use of nutritional supplements, herbal supplements, vitamins, and minerals
- Use of alcohol, caffeine, and nicotine

NURSING INTERVENTIONS

- Monitor food intake.
- Monitor fluid intake and output.
- Use client-centered approach to address disease-specific problems with ingestion, digestion, or medication regime. Qpcc
- Collaborate with dietitian. Qtc
- Provide adequate calories and high-quality protein.

STRATEGIES TO INCREASE PROTEIN, CALORIC CONTENT
- Add skim milk powder to milk (double-strength milk).
- Use whole milk instead of water in recipes.
- Add cheese, peanut butter, chopped hard-boiled eggs, or yogurt to foods.
- Dip meats in eggs or milk and coat with breadcrumbs before cooking.
- Nuts and dried beans are significant sources of protein. These are good alternatives for a dairy allergy or lactose intolerance.

Application Exercises

1. A nurse is discussing how the body uses nutrients for energy with a client during a primary care visit. Match each substance with the statement that describes how the body stores or processes it for energy.

   A. Glucose

   B. ATP

   C. Amino acids

   D. Fatty acids

   1. Converted to glycogen and stored in liver and muscle tissue

   2. Converted to triglycerides and stored in adipose tissue

   3. Used to synthesize proteins

   4. Used before glycogen and stored fat for growth and repair

2. A charge nurse is conducting a nutritional class for a group of newly licensed nurses regarding basal metabolic rate (BMR). Sort each factor by whether the nurse will discuss it as a factor that increases BMR or decreases BMR.

   A. Lactation

   B. Prolonged stress

   C. Hypothyroidism

   D. Puberty

   E. Age older than 60 years

3. A nurse is reviewing prescribed medications for newly admitted clients. Which do the nurse recognize as types of medications that decrease the BMR? (Select all that apply.)

   A. Epinephrine

   B. Levothyroxine

   C. Opioid

   D. Barbiturate

   E. Ephedrine sulfate

4. A nurse is caring for a client with negative nitrogen balance. Which of the following does the nurse recognize as possible causes of negative nitrogen balance? (Select all that apply.)

   A. Critical illness

   B. Starvation

   C. Adolescence

   D. Trauma

   E. Pregnancy

Active Learning Scenario

A nurse is conducting a nutritional program for a group of newly licensed nurses regarding how the body uses food for energy. Use the ATI Active Learning Template: Basic Concept to complete this item.

RELATED CONTENT: Describe the steps of ingestion, digestion, and absorption.

UNDERLYING PRINCIPLES: Explain the two processes that occur during metabolism.

Active Learning Scenario Key

Using the ATI Active Learning Template: Basic Concept

RELATED CONTENT

- Ingestion is the process of taking in food by mouth into the digestive system.
- Digestion involves the breakdown of food into nutrients so they can be absorbed.
- Absorption is the process by which nutrients pass through the walls of the digestive system so they can be used by the body.

UNDERLYING PRINCIPLES

- Catabolism is the process by which food is broken down into small molecules to release heat and chemical energy.
- Anabolism is the formation of new body substances (tissue, bone).

Ⓝ *NCLEX® Connection: Physiologic Adaptation, Illness Management*

Application Exercises Key

1. A, 1; B, 4; C, 3; D, 2

   When taking actions, the nurse should explain that the liver converts unused glucose to glycogen and stores it in the liver and muscle tissue for later use. Excess fatty acids are converted into triglycerides and stored in adipose tissue. Amino acids are used to make body proteins. Body cells use ATP for growth and repair and use glycogen and stored fat if no ATP is available.

   Ⓝ *NCLEX® Connection: Health Promotion, Disease Prevention*

2. **INCREASES BMR**: A, B, D; **DECREASES BMR**: C, E

   When taking actions, the nurse will inform the newly licensed nurses that metabolic needs increase during lactation, the stress response, and puberty, so clients should consume higher calories from nutrient-dense foods during those times. Decreased thyroid function in hypothyroidism causes reduced cellular regulation and decreased BMR. Loss of muscle mass associated with aging decreases the BMR.

   Ⓝ *NCLEX® Connection: Health Promotion and Maintenance, Aging Process*

3. C, D **CORRECT:** When recognizing cues about medications that decrease the BMR, the nurse identifies that opioids and barbiturates have CNS-depressant actions, which slow metabolic processes.

   Ⓝ *NCLEX® Connection: Basic Care and Comfort, Nutrition and Oral Hydration*

4. A, B, D **CORRECT:** When recognizing cues about negative nitrogen balance, the nurse identifies that critical illnesses, starvation/malnutrition, and trauma are possible causes of protein catabolism occurring at a faster rate than protein synthesis.

   Ⓝ *NCLEX® Connection: Reduction of Risk Potential, System-Specific Assessments*

UNIT 1   PRINCIPLES OF NUTRITION

CHAPTER 3
Nutrition Assessment/ Data Collection

Nurses play a key role in assessing the nutritional needs of clients. Nurses monitor and intervene with clients requiring acute and chronic nutritional care. Nurses should consider and incorporate the family's nutritional habits into a client's individual plan of care. Nurses should take an active role in assessing and teaching community groups regarding nutrition.

A collaborative, interprofessional approach provides the best outcomes for the client. Providers and nurses collect physical assessment data, as well as serving as liaisons between the health care team and the dietitian. The Joint Commission (TJC) requires a nutrition screening within 24 hours of admission to an inpatient facility, with referral to a dietitian for clients at risk for malnutrition. Registered dietitians complete comprehensive nutritional assessments. Nurses monitor and evaluate interventions provided to clients. Qᴛᴄ

A client's physical appearance can be deceiving. A client who has a healthy weight and appearance can be malnourished. Cultural, social, and physical norms must be part of a client's assessment. Even with adequate client education, personal preferences can be an overriding factor to successful nutritional balance.

DIET HISTORY

A diet history is an assessment of usual foods, fluids, and supplements. The diet history is part of the nutrition screening performed using various settings to determine malnutrition issues. Components of the diet history include the following.

- Time, type, and amount of food eaten for breakfast, lunch, dinner, and snacks Qᴘᴄᴄ
- Time, type, and amount of fluids consumed throughout the day, including water, health drinks, coffee/tea, carbonated beverages, and beverages with caffeine
- Type, amount, and frequency of "special foods" (celebration foods, movie foods)
- Typical preparation of foods and fluids (coffee with sugar, fried foods)
- Number of meals eaten away from home (at work or school)
- Type of preferred or prescribed diet (ovo-lacto vegetarian, 2 g sodium/low-fat diet)
- Foods avoided due to allergy or preference
- Frequency and dose/amount of medications or nutritional supplements taken daily
- Satisfaction with diet over a specified time frame (last 3 months, 1 year)

TOOLS TO DETERMINE NUTRITIONAL STATUS

A physical assessment is performed by the provider or nurse to identify indicators of inadequate nutrition. However, other diseases or conditions can cause these clinical findings.

MANIFESTATIONS
- Hair that is dry or brittle, or skin that has dry patches
- Poor wound healing or sores
- Lack of subcutaneous fat or muscle wasting
- Irregular cardiovascular measurements (heart rate and rhythm, blood pressure)
- Enlarged spleen or liver
- General weakness or impaired coordination

ANTHROPOMETRIC TOOLS

Weight
- Weigh at the same time of day wearing similar clothing to ensure accurate weight readings.
- Daily fluctuations generally are indicative of water weight changes.
- Percentage weight change calculation (weight change over a specified time):

$$\% \text{ weight change} = \frac{(\text{usual weight} - \text{present weight})}{\text{usual weight}} \times 100$$

- Ideal body weight based on the Hamwi method (also called Rule of 6 for males and Rule of 5 for females) using height/weight calculation.
  - **MALES:** 48 kg (106 lb) for the first 152 cm (5 ft) of height, and 2.7 kg (6 lb) for each additional 2.5 cm (1 in).
  - **FEMALES:** 45 kg (100 lb) for the first 152 cm (5 ft) of height, and 2.3 kg (5 lb) for each additional 2.5 cm (1 in).
- During illness, weight loss is monitored to prevent or detect malnutrition.
  - With starvation or chronic disease, weight loss indicating severe malnutrition: greater than 5%/month, greater than 7.5%/3 months, greater than 10%/6 months, greater than 20%/year
  - With acute disease or injury, weight loss indicating severe malnutrition: greater than 2%/week, greater than 5%/month, greater than 7.5%/3 months

Height

- Measure on a vertical, flat surface. Ask the client to remove shoes and head coverings and stand straight with heels together looking straight ahead. Read the measurement to the nearest 0.1 cm or 1/8 inch.
- Obtain a recumbent measurement (lying on a firm, flat surface) for infants and young children.

Body mass index (BMI)

BMI measurements compare the weight to height to estimate the effect of the individual's body weight. Client factors should be considered when determining the value of BMI measurement. For example, a client who has large muscle mass compared to height can have an increased BMI, since weight can be influenced by both fat and muscle, or a client with a normal BMI might have excess body fat.

- Healthy weight is indicated by a BMI of 18.5 to 24.9.
- Underweight is indicated by a BMI less than 18.5.
- Overweight is defined as an increased body weight in relation to height. It is indicated by a BMI of 25 to 29.9, and are about 20% above desirable levels.
- Obesity is indicated by a BMI greater than or equal to 30.

$$BMI = weight (kg) \div height (m^2)$$

CLINICAL VALUES

Fluid I&O

- Adults: 2,000 to 3,000 mL (2 to 3 L) per day
- Total average output: 1,750 to 3,000 mL/day

Protein levels are usually measured by albumin levels, although total protein is sometimes used.

- Many non-nutritional factors (injury, kidney disease), interfere with this measure for protein malnutrition.
- Expected reference range for albumin: 3.5 to 5 g/dL

Prealbumin (thyroxine-binding protein) is a sensitive measure used to assess critically ill clients who are at risk for malnutrition. This test reflects acute changes rather than gradual changes. However, it is more expensive and often unavailable. This is not part of routine assessment.

- Prealbumin levels can decrease with an inflammatory process resulting in an inaccurate measurement.
- Prealbumin levels are used to measure effectiveness of total parenteral nutrition.
- Expected reference range is 15 to 36 mg/dL. (Less than 10.7 mg/dL indicates severe nutritional deficiency.)

Nitrogen balance refers to the relationship between protein breakdown (catabolism) and protein synthesis (anabolism).

- To measure nitrogen balance
  - Record protein intake (g) over 24 hr and divide by 6.25.
    - 24 hr protein intake ÷ 6.25 = nitrogen intake (g)
  - Record nitrogen excretion in urine over 24 hr and add 4 g.
    - 24 hr urinary urea nitrogen + 4 g = total nitrogen output
  - Subtract nitrogen output from nitrogen intake.

Nitrogen intake − total nitrogen output = nitrogen balance

- A neutral nitrogen balance indicates adequate nutritional intake.
- A positive nitrogen balance indicates protein synthesis is greater than protein breakdown as during growth, pregnancy, or during recovery.
- A negative nitrogen balance indicates protein is used at a greater rate than it is synthesized as in starvation or a catabolic state following injury or disease.

RISK FACTORS FOR INADEQUATE NUTRITION

BIOPHYSICAL FACTORS

- Medical disease/conditions (hypertension, HIV/AIDS)
- Preventive measures or disease treatments, including surgery or use of medications and supplements.
- Genetic predisposition (lactose intolerance, osteoporosis)
- Age

PSYCHOLOGICAL FACTORS

- Mental illness (clinical depression)
- Excessive stress
- Negative self-concept
- Use of comfort foods

SOCIAL DETERMINANTS OF HEALTH ○SDoH

NEIGHBORHOOD AND BUILT ENVIRONMENT

- Pollutants in air, soil, water cause risks to food supply
- Limited options for food in community affect nutritious food choices
- Limited transportation methods affect ability to transport groceries

SOCIAL AND COMMUNITY CONTEXT
- Food preparation methods may increase likelihood of food-borne illnesses.
- Unstable living situation leads to inconsistent food supply.
- Health education materials may not include cultural food preferences.

ECONOMIC STABILITY
- May have to choose between quality foods and housing or educational expenses
- Lack of health insurance impacts ability to consult with dietitian.
- Lack of affordable, nutritious food may lead to undernutrition or overnutrition.

FOOD AND NUTRITION:
- Availability of food and nutrients
- Access to healthy food options
- Reliable sources of food

HEALTH AND HEALTH CARE
- Lack of primary care resources limits follow-up for chronic conditions associated with obesity
- Limited number of school nurses affects screening for nutritional deficits.
- Lack of access to telehealth resources for nutrition consults.

EDUCATION
- Literacy levels affect ability to read food labels
- Education level affects ability to earn wages consistent with cost of living.
- Education level affects ability to problem-solve and make healthy food choices.

EFFECT OF RISK FACTORS ON NUTRITIONAL STATUS

The following are examples of how risk factors can affect nutritional status.
- A client who has edema can require treatment with a diuretic and low-sodium diet. Diuretics can cause sodium and potassium imbalances. A low-sodium diet can be unappetizing and cause the client to eat less.
- Osteoporosis has many modifiable risk factors. A client who takes action to prevent osteoporosis (increasing intake of vitamin D and calcium, engaging in weight-bearing exercise, reducing use of tobacco and alcohol products) will positively affect their nutritional status.
- Poor self-concept can cause a client to avoid eating or to overeat.

NURSING ACTIONS
- In addition to determining the client's nutrient and calorie intake, assess other factors that might alter nutrient intake.
- Consult with the provider to see if the client's medical treatment plan needs to be altered to improve nutrition, such as administering a different medication to prevent the adverse effect of anorexia or adding a medication to treat nausea or improve appetite.
- Plan the client's schedule of activities to prevent interruptions during mealtime, and to avoid fatigue, nausea, or pain before meals.

Application Exercises

1. A nurse is caring for a client who is malnourished. Describe manifestations the nurse should expect to find on physical examination.

2. A nurse in a nutrition clinic is calculating body mass index (BMI) for several clients. The nurse should identify which of the following client BMIs as overweight?
   A. 24
   B. 30
   C. 27
   D. 32

3. A nurse on an orthopedic unit is reviewing data for a client who sustained trauma in a motor-vehicle crash. Which of the following values indicates the client is in a catabolic state (using protein faster than protein is being synthesized)?
   A. Blood albumin 3.5 g/dL
   B. Negative nitrogen balance
   C. BMI of 18.5
   D. Blood prealbumin 15 mg/dL

4. A nurse is caring for a client who has risk factors for nutritional deficits related to social determinants of health (SDOH). Match the risk factor with the SDOH category in which it best fits.

A. No grocery stores in community	1. Education
B. Family members discourage asking for help	2. Neighborhood and built environment
C. Inability to afford health insurance	3. Economic stability
D. No access to primary care	4. Health and health care
E. Low level of literacy	5. Social and community context

5. A nurse is teaching a group of clients about risk factors for developing osteoporosis. Which of the following risk factors should the nurse include? (Select all that apply.)
   A. Inactivity
   B. Family history
   C. BMI 30 or greater
   D. Hyperlipidemia
   E. Cigarette smoking

Active Learning Scenario

A community health nurse is conducting a dietary assessment for a client. Use the ATI Active Learning Template: Basic Concept to complete this item.

UNDERLYING PRINCIPLES: Describe four components of a diet history.

Active Learning Scenario Key

Using the ATI Active Learning Template: Basic Concept

UNDERLYING PRINCIPLES: A diet history is an assessment of usual foods, fluids, and supplements.

- Time, type, and amount of food eaten for breakfast, lunch, dinner, and snacks.
- Time, type, and amount of fluids consumed throughout the day including water, health drinks, coffee/tea, carbonated beverages, and beverages with caffeine.
- Type, amount, and frequency of "special foods" (celebration foods, movie foods).
- Typical preparation of foods and fluids (coffee with sugar, fried foods).
- Number of meals eaten away from home (at work or school).
- Type of diet (ovo-lacto vegetarian, 2 g sodium/low-fat diet).
- Foods avoided due to allergy or preference.
- Frequency and dose/amount of medications or nutritional supplements taken daily.
- Satisfaction with diet over a specified time frame (last 3 months, year).

Ⓝ *NCLEX® Connection: Health Promotion and Maintenance, Health Screening*

Application Exercises Key

1. When recognizing cues with a client who is malnourished, the nurse should expect to find manifestations that include but are not limited to: poor wound healing; dry hair, dry skin, dry nails; weak hand grip strength; impaired coordination; depression; swollen lymph nodes in the neck and cheeks; heart rate or rhythm not within expected ranges; blood pressure not within expected range; decreased balance and coordination; enlarged liver or spleen; and edema of the lower extremities.

   Ⓝ *NCLEX® Connection: Basic Care and Comfort, Nutrition and Oral Hydration*

2. C. **CORRECT:** When recognizing cues, the nurse should identify a BMI in the range of 25 to 29.9 as overweight, an increased body weight in relation to height..

   Ⓝ *NCLEX® Connection: Basic Care and Comfort, Nutrition and Oral Hydration*

3. B. **CORRECT:** When recognizing cues, the nurse identifies that negative nitrogen balance indicates protein is used at a greater rate than it is synthesized, as in starvation or a catabolic state following injury or disease.

   Ⓝ *NCLEX® Connection: Reduction of Risk Potential, Laboratory Values*

4. A, 2; B, 5; C, 3; D, 4; E, 1

   When recognizing cues, the nurse should identify the lack of grocery stores in the community as an SDOH that affects nutritious food supply in the neighborhood and built environment. The nurse should identify family members discouraging the client from asking for help as a social and community context SDOH. The nurse should identify inability to afford health insurance as an SDOH related to economic stability. The nurse should identify a low level of literacy as an SDOH related to education that affects the ability to read educational materials or food labels.

   Ⓝ *NCLEX® Connection: Health Promotion and Maintenance, Health Promotion/Disease Prevention*

5. A, B. E. **CORRECT:** When taking the action of teaching clients about risk factors for developing osteoporosis, the nurse should identify that inactivity, family history, and cigarette smoking are all factors that increase the risk for developing osteoporosis.

   Ⓝ *NCLEX® Connection: Health Promotion and Maintenance, Health Promotion/Disease Prevention*

UNIT 1 PRINCIPLES OF NUTRITION

CHAPTER 4 *Guidelines for Healthy Eating*

Nutrition is vital to maintaining optimal health. Healthy food choices and controlling weight are important steps in promoting health and reducing risk factors for disease.

Nurses should encourage favorable nutritional choices and can serve as informational resources for clients regarding guidelines for healthy eating.

Established guidelines for healthy eating that clients and nurses can refer to include the Dietary Guidelines for Americans and MyPlate, along with several condition- or system-specific guidelines.

Vegetarian diets can meet all nutrient recommendations. It is essential to consume a variety and correct portions of foods to meet individual caloric needs.

DIETARY GUIDELINES FOR AMERICANS

- The U.S. Department of Agriculture (USDA) and the U.S. Department of Health and Human Services (HHS) publish the Dietary Guidelines for Americans jointly every 5 years. These guidelines are based on evidence-based advice concerning food intake and physical activity for Americans. The new 2020-2025 guidelines are the first edition that provide recommendations by life stage beginning with birth and continuing through older adulthood. The updates can be found on the USDA and health.gov websites.
- The Dietary Guidelines for Americans advocates healthy food selections: a variety of fiber-rich fruits and vegetables, whole grains, low-fat or fat-free milk and milk products, lean meats, poultry, fish, legumes, eggs, and nuts. Recommendations include nutrient-dense foods and beverages. The 2020-2025 Guidelines provide four overarching Guidelines to encourage healthy eating patterns for each stage of life

- Follow a healthy dietary pattern at every stage of life
  - For about the first 6 months of life, exclusively feed infants human milk or iron-fortified infant formula if human milk is not available. Provide supplemental vitamin D beginning soon after birth.
  - At about 6 months, introduce nutrient-dense complimentary food that include a variety of foods from all food groups.
  - From 12 months through older adulthood, follow a healthy dietary pattern that meets nutrient needs, achieves a healthy body weight, and reduces the risk of developing chronic disease.
- Customize and enjoy nutrient-dense food and beverage choices to reflect personal preferences, cultural traditions, and budgetary considerations.
  - The Dietary Guidelines provide a framework that is designed for customization for individual needs and preferences as well as foodways of diverse cultures.
- Focus on meeting food group needs with nutrient-dense foods and beverages and stay within calorie limits.
  - Core elements of a healthy dietary pattern include:
    - Vegetables of all types (dark green; red and orange; beans, peas, and lentils; starchy; and other vegetables)
    - Fruits (especially whole fruits)
    - Grains (at least half should be whole grain)
    - Dairy (fat-free or low-fat milk, yogurt and cheese or alternatives if needed)
    - Protein foods (lean meats, poultry, and eggs; seafood; beans, peas, and lentils; nuts, seeds, and soy products)
    - Oils (vegetable oils and oils in foods such as seafood and nuts)
- Limit foods and beverages with high amounts of added sugars, saturated fat, and sodium.
  - Foods and beverages high in added sugars, saturated fat, or sodium as well as alcoholic beverages should be limited.
    - Added sugars: Starting at age 2, less than 10% of cal/day. For those younger than age 2, avoid foods and beverages with added sugars.
    - Saturated fat: Choose monounsaturated and polyunsaturated fats from fish, lean meats, nuts, and vegetable oils. Starting at age 2, limit to less than 10% of cal/day.
    - Sodium: Less than 2,300 mg/day (about 1 tsp) of salt. Limit canned and processed foods. Prepare foods without adding salt.
    - Alcoholic beverages: Drinking less is better for health. If choosing to drink alcohol, drink in moderation by limiting intake to 2 drinks or less per day for men and 1 drink or less in a day for women.

- General Dietary Recommendations for Adults, based on the Dietary Guidelines for Americans
  - Recommendations are based on a 2,000-calorie daily diet.
  - Vegetables – 2 1/2 cups per day, including a variety throughout the week:
    - Green vegetables
    - Orange and red vegetables
    - Starchy vegetables
    - Peas and lentils
  - Fruits – 2 cups per day
  - Grains – 6 ounces per day, including more than 3 ounces of whole grains
  - Dairy – 3 cups per day
  - Protein – 5 1/2; cups per day, including:
    - Poultry and other meats
    - Eggs
    - Seafood
    - Soy, nuts, seeds
  - Oils – 27 grams per day
- The Dietary Guidelines for Americans also establishes recommendations for age groups:
  - Toddlers ages 12 through 23 months who are no longer receiving human milk or infant formula
  - Children ages 2 through 8
  - Children and adolescents ages 9 through 13
  - Adolescents ages 14 through 18
  - Adults ages 19 through 59
  - Women who are pregnant or lactating
  - Adults ages 60 and older
- Follow food safety guidelines when preparing, cooking, and storing food. Avoid consumption of raw eggs and unpasteurized milk and juices. **Qs**
  - These strategies are beneficial for cooking foods at home.
    - When using convenience foods or boxed meals, add healthy ingredients (frozen vegetables, canned legumes) to increase the volume of food and add nutrition.
    - Decrease the amount of salt or seasonings containing sodium when cooking.
    - Buy side items that increase the nutritional value of meals (packaged salad kits, pre-cut fruit, whole-grain bread).
  - When eating out, these strategies can help meet nutritional guidelines.
    - Eat a snack with high-fiber content 1 hour before the restaurant meal to decrease hunger.
    - If restaurant meal will be high-calorie, eat lower calorie, nutrient-dense foods for other meals that day.
    - Ask for items with high fat content on the side (for example, dressings, sauces, gravies, creams)
    - Base restaurant choices on those that offer healthy options.

PHYSICAL ACTIVITY

Physical activity is one of the most important things an individual can do to improve their overall health status. Establish exercise routines to promote cardiovascular health, muscle strength and endurance, and psychological well-being.

Benefits of physical activity start accumulating with small amounts and activity and immediately after completing activity.

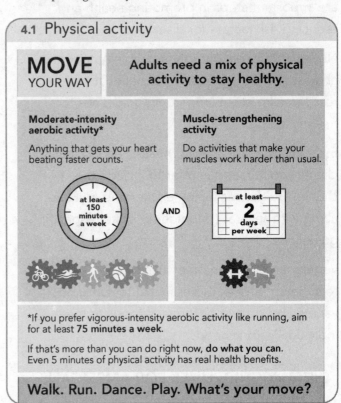

4.1 Physical activity

MOVE YOUR WAY

Adults need a mix of physical activity to stay healthy.

Moderate-intensity aerobic activity*

Anything that gets your heart beating faster counts.

at least 150 minutes a week

AND

Muscle-strengthening activity

Do activities that make your muscles work harder than usual.

at least 2 days per week

*If you prefer vigorous-intensity aerobic activity like running, aim for at least **75 minutes a week.**

If that's more than you can do right now, **do what you can.** Even 5 minutes of physical activity has real health benefits.

Walk. Run. Dance. Play. What's your move?

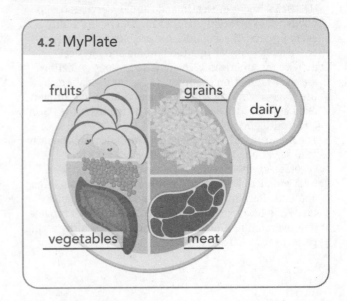

4.2 MyPlate

fruits | grains

dairy

vegetables | meat

MYPLATE

The USDA sponsors a website that promotes healthy food choices balanced with physical activity (www.myPlate.gov). MyPlate is based on the current USDA dietary guidelines and is a tool to help individuals identify daily amounts of foods based on criteria (age, sex, activity level). The food groups represented are grains, vegetables, fruits, dairy, and protein foods.

- MyPlate can serve as a reminder to balance calorie intake with suitable activity.
- Multiple resources are available such as MyPlate Kitchen, where a client can find recipes and resources within the kitchen and ideas for healthy eating tips on a budget.
- The MyPlate website offers age-and lifestyle-specific information and resources for women during pregnancy and lactation. Resources are available for the older adult population.
- The MyPlate image and information sheet are available in multiple languages to assist with client education.

VEGETARIAN DIETS

- A vegetarian diet focuses on plants for food, including fruits, vegetables, dried beans and peas, grains, seeds, and nuts. There is no single type of vegetarian diet. Vegetarian eating patterns usually fall into the following groups.
  - **Vegan** diet excludes all meat and animal products.
  - **Raw vegan diet** is a strictly uncooked food eating pattern based on fruit, vegetables, nuts, seeds, legumes, and sprouted grains. Uncooked food ranges from 75% to 100% of total food consumed
  - **Lacto vegetarian** diet includes dairy products.
  - **Lacto-ovo vegetarian** diet includes dairy products and eggs.
- People who follow vegetarian diets can get all the nutrients they need, but they must be careful to eat a wide variety of foods to meet their nutritional needs. It is important to discuss ensuring enough vitamin D and B12, calcium, and omega-3 fatty acids are consumed by clients who follow a vegan diet.
- Vegetarian diets and eating patterns can be beneficial and can reduce the risk and aid in the treatment of certain health conditions including ischemic heart disease, type 2 diabetes, and certain cancers.

FOOD LABELS

- The Food and Drug Administration (FDA) requires certain information be included with packaged foods and beverages. The information is included on the nutrition facts label or food label, which is a boxed label found on foods and beverages. Food labels must include the name and form of the product, the net amount of the food or beverage by weight, measure, or count, and the name and address of the manufacturer, packer, or distributor.
- The Percent Daily Values information is typically based on a 2,000 calorie/day diet
- The label must contain the ingredient list and the foods must be listed in descending order by weight.
- Multiple changes have been made to food labels to reflect how individuals currently eat and drink

NUTRIENTS INCLUDED ON THE FOOD LABEL
Actual amounts of nutrients declared, not just the % daily value
- Calories (in larger bold type)
- Total fat
- Saturated fat
- Trans fat
- Cholesterol
- Sodium
- Total carbohydrates
- Dietary fiber
- Sugars (included in grams and as a % daily value)
- Protein
- Vitamin D
- Potassium
- Calcium
- Iron
- Manufacturers are required to clearly state if a food product contains any of the eight allergens that are responsible for 90% of all food allergies (milk, eggs, fish, crustacean shellfish, tree nuts, peanuts, wheat, soybeans).
- Foods marketed as functional foods might be whole foods or foods with additives (herbs, minerals). These foods are often advertised as having the ability to prevent or promote disease. There are currently no regulations regarding functional foods.
- Organic food products are regulated under the USDA.
  - Organic foods are produced without the use of pesticides or synthetic fertilizer.
  - Organic livestock must have the ability to graze on pastures, are fed 100% organic feed, and do not receive hormones, or antibiotics.
- Organic foods can reduce the risk of pathogen resistance to antibiotics. While they reduce exposure to pesticides, there is no evidence that it has a healthy effect. Clarify misinformation about these foods with clients.

CLIENT EDUCATION
- Read food labels properly (comparing nutrient, calorie, fat, and sodium levels) to ensure individual nutritional needs are met, and healthy choices are made.
- Goods that are genetically engineered or contain genetically modified organisms (GMO) have not been proven harmful.

STRATEGIES FOR PROMOTION OF SPECIFIC AREAS OF HEALTH

Heart

- Limit saturated fat to 7% of calories.
- Limit intake of red and processed meats, refined grains, added sugars, butter, high sodium foods, and commercial trans-fat.
- Consume a diet higher in fiber, vitamins, antioxidants, mineral, polynutrients, and unsaturated fat and lower in glycemic index.
- The Dietary Approaches to Stop Hypertension (DASH) diet is proven by research to significantly lower systolic and diastolic blood pressure as well as low-density lipoprotein cholesterol. Q EBP

Neurologic system

- Normal functioning of the neurologic system depends on adequate levels of the B-complex vitamins, especially thiamin (B1), biotin, and vitamins B_6 and B_{12}.
- Calcium and sodium are important regulators of nerve responses. Consuming the recommended servings from the grain and dairy food groups provides these nutrients.

Bones

- Consuming the recommended servings from the MyPlate's dairy group supplies the calcium, magnesium, and phosphorus necessary for bone formation.
- Weight-bearing physical activity is essential to decrease the risk of osteoporosis.

Bowel function

- Normal bowel functioning depends on adequate fluid intake and 25 g/day of fiber for females, and 38 g/day for males.
- The minimum number of servings from MyPlate's fruit, vegetable, and grain food groups (specifically whole grains) provides the essential nutrients.

Cancer prevention

- A well-balanced diet using MyPlate and a healthy weight are guidelines to prevent cancer.
- Increase high-fiber, plant-based foods.
- Limit saturated and trans fat, while emphasizing foods with polyunsaturated fats (omega-3 fatty acids).
- Limit sodium intake.
- Avoid excess alcohol intake.
- Include regular physical activity.

Active Learning Scenario

A community health nurse is conducting a nutritional class regarding cancer prevention strategies. Use the ATI Active Learning Template: Basic Concept to complete this item.

RELATED CONTENT: Describe four components recommended to prevent cancer.

Application Exercises

1. A nurse is conducting a nutrition class at a local community center. Which of the following information should the nurse include in the teaching?

   A. Limit saturated fat to less than 10% of total daily intake.

   B. Good bowel function requires 35 g/day of fiber for females.

   C. Depends on B-Limit cholesterol consumption to 400 mg/day.

   D. Normal functioning cardiac systems depend on B-Complex vitamins.

2. A nurse is providing teaching to a client who follows vegan dietary practices. The nurse should instruct the client that there is a risk of having a deficit in which of the following nutrients? (Select all that apply.)

   A. Vitamin D

   B. Fiber

   C. Calcium

   D. Vitamin B_{12}

   E. Whole grains

3. A school nurse is teaching a group of students how to read food labels. Which of the following is a required component of food labels that the nurse should include in the teaching? (Select all that apply.)

   A. Total carbohydrates

   B. Total fat

   C. Calories

   D. Magnesium

   E. Dietary fiber

4. A nurse is discussing essential nutrients for normal functioning of the nervous system with a client. Which of the following should the nurse include in the teaching? (Select all that apply.)

   A. Calcium

   B. Thiamin

   C. Vitamin B_6

   D. Sodium

   E. Phosphorus

Application Exercises Key

1. A. **CORRECT:** When taking actions and teaching about nutrition to clients, the nurse should include for the clients to limit saturated fat to less than 10% of total daily intake.

(N) *NCLEX® Connection: Health Promotion and Maintenance, Health Promotion/Disease Prevention*

2. A. **CORRECT:** When taking actions, the nurse should Instruct the client to ensure an adequate consumption of vitamin D because most dietary vitamin D is consumed via fortified milk products. The vegan diet includes plant foods and excludes all animal-derived products.
   C. **CORRECT:** Instruct the client to monitor and ensure an adequate consumption of calcium because there are few good sources of calcium from plant sources.
   D. **CORRECT:** The nurse should also teach the client to ensure they are consuming adequate vitamin B_{12} because all reliable sources of vitamin B_{12} are in animal products.

(N) *NCLEX® Connection: Health Promotion and Maintenance, Health Promotion/Disease Prevention*

3. A, B, C, E. **CORRECT:** When taking actions and teaching about how to read food labels, the school should teach the students that The Food and Drug Administration (FDA) requires certain information be included with packaged foods and beverages. Total carbohydrates, single serving size, number of servings in the package, percent of daily values, and the amount of each nutrient in one serving are all required elements. Total fat is included on food labels as well as calories and dietary fiber.

(N) *NCLEX® Connection: Health Promotion and Maintenance, Aging Process*

4. A, D. **CORRECT:** When taking actions and discussing essential nutrients for normal functioning of the neurologic system, the nurse should include calcium and sodium are important regulators of nerve responses.
   B, C. **CORRECT:** The nurse should also include that normal function requires adequate levels of the B-complex vitamins, (especially thiamin, biotin, and vitamins B_6 and B_{12}).

(N) *NCLEX® Connection: Health Promotion and Maintenance, Health Promotion/Disease Prevention*

Active Learning Scenario Key

Using the ATI Active Learning Template: Basic Concept
RELATED CONTENT

A well-balanced diet using the MyPlate and a healthy weight are guidelines to prevent cancer.
- Increase high-fiber plant-based foods.
- Limit saturated and polyunsaturated fat while emphasizing foods with monounsaturated fat or omega-3 fatty acids (nuts and fish).
- Limit sodium intake.
- Avoid excess alcohol intake.
- Include regular physical activity.

(N) *NCLEX® Connection: Health Promotion and Maintenance, Health Promotion/Disease Prevention*

UNIT 1   PRINCIPLES OF NUTRITION

CHAPTER 5   *Food Safety*

Food safety is an important concept in nursing. It is essential to provide clients with the necessary education regarding food safety and food-medication interactions.

Food safety concerns include preventing aspiration of food, reducing the risk of foodborne illness, assessing for food allergies, and understanding food-medication interactions.

FOOD SAFETY GUIDELINES

Ingestion of food poses a risk of aspiration in some circumstances.
- To minimize the risk of aspiration, food should be consumed only by individuals who are conscious and have an intact gag or swallow reflex. Qs
- For clients who have a known risk of aspiration (following a stroke or a procedure involving anesthesia of the esophagus), it is important for nurses to monitor the client's ability to swallow prior to eating.
- Young children are at an increased risk for aspiration of some foods.

FOOD SAFETY REQUIREMENTS
- Proper food storage
- Proper handling
- Proper preparation

FOOD STORAGE GUIDELINES

Fresh meat: Maintain refrigerator temperature at 40° F (4° C) or colder.
- **Bacon**: 7 days
- **Sausage** (pork/chicken/beef/turkey): 1 to 2 days
- **Summer sausage**: 3 months (unopened); 3 weeks (opened)
- **Steaks, chops, roasts** (beef, veal, lamb, or pork): 3 to 5 days
- **Chicken or turkey** (whole/parts): 1 to 2 days
- **Fish**: Maintain refrigerator temperature at 40° F (4° C) or colder.
  - Lean or fatty: 1 to 2 days
  - Smoked: 14 days
  - Fresh shellfish: 1 to 2 days
  - Canned: 3 to 4 days (after opening); 5 years (pantry)

Eggs: Store in the refrigerator for 3 to 5 weeks in shell, and 1 week if hard-boiled.

Fruits and vegetables: Refrigerate perishable fruits and vegetables at 40° F (4° C). All pre-cut and pre-peeled fruits and vegetables should also be refrigerated.

Perishables: Do not leave at room temperature for more than 2 hr (1 hr if the temperature is 90° F [32° C] or above).

Canned goods: Check for rusting, crushing, and denting. Observe for stickiness on the outside of can, which can indicate leakage. Do not use any canned foods that are damaged.

HANDLING GUIDELINES

- Wash hands and food preparation surfaces frequently, and before handling food.
- Separate foods to avoid cross-contamination.

PREPARATION GUIDELINES

Cook food to the proper temperature followed by a 3-min rest time.
- Roasts and steaks: 145° F (63° C)
- Chicken: 165° F (74° C)
- Ground beef: 160° F (71° C)
- Products that contain eggs: 160° F (71° C)

PACKAGING LABELS
- **Sell-by date**: The final recommended day of sale.
- **Use-by date:** How long the product will maintain top quality.
- **Expiration date**: The final day the product should be used or consumed.

FOODBORNE ILLNESS

Foodborne illnesses occur due to improper storage of food products, as well as unsafe handling and preparation. To decrease the incidence of foodborne illnesses, primary education should be conducted by nurses. Proper handing and preparation are simple and include performing frequent hand hygiene. It is important to refrigerate food products when necessary, and to avoid cross-contamination when preparing food. Food should be heated to recommended temperatures to kill unwanted bacteria. Following these basic principles can prevent the occurrence of foodborne illnesses. Qs
- Foodborne illnesses pose the greatest risk to children, older adults, immunocompromised clients, and pregnant clients.
- Viruses cause most foodborne illnesses, but bacteria are responsible for most deaths caused by foodborne illness.
- Foods most associated with foodborne illness are the following.
  - Raw or undercooked foods of animal origin
  - Raw fruits and vegetables contaminated with animal feces
  - Raw sprouts
  - Unpasteurized fruit juice and milk products
  - Uncooked food handled by someone who is ill

COMMON FOODBORNE ILLNESSES

Bacterial

Salmonella: Occurs due to eating undercooked or raw meat, poultry, eggs, fish, fruit, and dairy products. Common manifestations include headache, fever, abdominal cramping, diarrhea, nausea, and vomiting. This condition can be fatal.

Escherichia coli 0157:H7 Raw or undercooked meat, especially ground beef, can cause this foodborne pathogen. Findings include severe abdominal pain and diarrhea. The pathogen can also cause hemolytic uremic syndrome, which manifests as severe anemia and kidney failure.

Listeria monocytogenes: Soft cheese, raw milk products, undercooked poultry, processed meats, and raw vegetables can cause this illness. Listeria monocytogenes causes significant problems for newborns, pregnant clients, and immunocompromised clients. Onset occurs with the development of a sudden fever, diarrhea, headache, back pain, and abdominal discomfort. It can lead to stillbirth or miscarriage.

Viral

Norovirus: A viral infection caused by consuming contaminated fruits and vegetables, salads prepared by someone who is infected, oysters, and contaminated water. Norovirus is very contagious and has an onset of 24 to 48 hr. Manifestations include projectile vomiting, fever, myalgia, watery diarrhea, and headache.

FOOD ALLERGIES

Nutritional assessment/data collection includes identification of food allergies. A food allergy is a reaction that will occur each time the client is exposed to the food and initiate release of serotonin and histamine. Food intolerances do not occur consistently and are dependent on the amount of food eaten.

- Milk, peanuts, fish, eggs, soy, shellfish, tree nuts, and wheat are the most reported food allergies in adults. Some infants exhibit an allergic reaction to cow's milk and/or soy, but typically outgrow this by 4 years of age.
- Common manifestations of food allergy include nausea, vomiting, diarrhea, abdominal distention, and pain. Some reactions are severe and can cause.

FOOD-MEDICATION INTERACTIONS

Foods and medications can interact in the body in ways that alter the intended action of medications. The composition and timing of food intake should be considered in relation to medication use.

Foods can alter the absorption of medications.
- **Increased absorption**: Improves the peak effects of some drugs when taken with food.
- **Decreased absorption**: Food can decrease the rate and extent of absorption.
- Reducing the rate of absorption delays the onset of peak effects.
- Reducing the extent of absorption reduces the intended effect of the medication.

Some medications cause gastric irritation. It is important to take those medications (ibuprofen, amoxicillin, some antidepressants [bupropion]) with food to avoid gastric upset.

Some foods alter the metabolism/actions of medications. Qs
- Grapefruit juice interferes with the metabolism of many medications, resulting in an increased blood level of the medication.
- Foods high in vitamin K (dark green vegetables, eggs, carrots) can decrease the anticoagulant effects of warfarin.
- Foods high in protein can increase the metabolism of the anti-Parkinson's medication levodopa, which decreases the medication's absorption and amount transported to the brain.
- Tyramine is a naturally occurring amine found in many foods that has hypertensive effects like other amines (norepinephrine). Tyramine is metabolized by MAO, and clients taking MAOIs (phenelzine, selegiline) who consume foods high in tyramine can suffer a hypertensive crisis. Foods high in tyramine include aged cheese, smoked meats, dried fish, and overripe avocados.
- Herbal supplements can cause potential interactions with prescribed medications. It is important that any herbal medication consumed by a client be discussed with the provider.

NURSING ASSESSMENT/DATA COLLECTION AND INTERVENTIONS

- Nursing assessments should include a complete dietary profile of the client, medications, herbal supplements, baseline knowledge about food safety, and food-medication interactions.
- Nursing interventions should include basic teaching about food safety, and the interactions between food and client medications.
- Teach the client about the difference between food intolerance and food allergy.

Application Exercises

1. A nurse is teaching about norovirus to a group of adults at a local community center. Which of the following information should the nurse include?

   A. Use of hand sanitizer when handling foods will protect against norovirus.

   B. Clients who are pregnant are more susceptible to developing norovirus.

   C. Norovirus usually lasts 4 to 5 days.

   D. The onset of norovirus is 24 to 48 hours after exposure to the pathogen.

2. A nurse is providing teaching about food allergies to a group of new parents. Infants who react to which of the following foods typically outgrow the sensitivity? (Select all that apply.)

   A. Soy

   B. Wheat

   C. Cow's milk

   D. Eggs

   E. Fish

3. A nurse is providing teaching to a client who is to begin taking the MAOI selegiline. Consuming which of the following foods while taking this medication could cause a hypertensive crisis?

   A. Grapefruit juice

   B. Dark green vegetables

   C. Greek yogurt

   D. Smoked fish

Active Learning Scenario

A nurse is providing teaching to a client about food-borne illnesses. What should the nurse include in the teaching? Use the ATI Active Learning Template: Basic Concept to complete this item.

UNDERLYING PRINCIPLES

• Describe three foodborne illnesses and how they are acquired

Application Exercises Key

1. D. **CORRECT:** When taking actions, the nurse should Include in the teaching that norovirus can develop after 24 to 48 hours after exposure to the virus.

   Ⓝ *NCLEX® Connection: Health Promotion and Maintenance, Aging Process*

2. A, C. **CORRECT:** When taking actions, the nurse should teach new parents that Infants who react to soy and cow's milk typically outgrow the sensitivity by the age of 4 years.

   Ⓝ *NCLEX® Connection: Health Promotion and Maintenance, Aging Process*

3. D. **CORRECT:** When taking actions, the nurse should teach the client that smoked fish is high in tyramine, which has hypertensive effects like other amines. Because tyramine is metabolized by MAO, clients who are taking MAOIs and consume tyramine can experience a hypertensive crisis.

   Ⓝ *NCLEX® Connection: Basic Care and Comfort, Nutrition and Oral Hydration*

Active Learning Scenario Key

Using the ATI Active Learning Template: Basic Concept

UNDERLYING PRINCIPLES

Foodborne illnesses

- Salmonella: Occurs due to eating undercooked or raw meat, poultry, eggs, fish, fruit, and dairy products. Common manifestations include headache, fever, abdominal cramping, diarrhea, nausea, and vomiting. This condition can be fatal.
- *Escherichia coli* 0157:H7: Raw or undercooked meat, especially ground beef, can cause this foodborne pathogen. Findings include severe abdominal pain and diarrhea.
- *Listeria monocytogenes*: Soft cheese, raw milk products, undercooked poultry, processed meats, and raw vegetables can cause the illness. Listeria monocytogenes causes significant problems for newborns, pregnant clients, and immunocompromised clients. Onset occurs with the development of a sudden fever, diarrhea, headache, back pain, and abdominal discomfort. It can lead to stillbirth or miscarriage.
- Norovirus: A viral infection caused by consuming contaminated fruits and vegetables, salads prepared by someone who is infected, oysters, and contaminated water. Norovirus is very contagious and has an onset of 24 to 48 hr. Manifestations include projectile vomiting, fever, myalgia, watery diarrhea, and headache.

Ⓝ *NCLEX® Connection: Health Promotion and Maintenance, Health Promotion/Disease Prevention*

UNIT 1   PRINCIPLES OF NUTRITION

CHAPTER 6 *Cultural, Ethnic, and Religious Influences*

Cultural, ethnic, and religious considerations greatly affect nutritional health. Understanding that ideas regarding food choices and nutrition vary among cultures can help to prevent ethnocentrism (identifying and incorporating individual preferences promotes client-centered care). Q︎PCC

Cultural traditions affect food choices and routines. Nurses should take this into consideration when planning and communicating nutritional goals with clients.

Acculturation is the process of a cultural, ethnic, or religious group's adopting of the dominant culture's behaviors, beliefs, and values. Q︎SDoH

Considering the client's foodway can be a helpful way to determine dietary preferences, which includes the role of foods, food preparation, what foods are considered edible, timing of meals, and use of food for health or other benefits.

CULTURE AND NUTRITION

- Culture influences every aspect of life, including nutritional intake. While common preferences exist within some cultures, individual preferences and the degree to which the client follows cultural recommendations can vary greatly. For further information on culture, refer to Fundamentals Chapter 35: Cultural and Spiritual Nursing Care.
- Food might be symbolic for a client.
  - Representing masculinity or femininity
  - Viewed as expressions of love or punishment
  - Representing connectedness or separateness
  - Part of celebration or mourning
  - "Comfort foods" that relate to a client's past
- Culture defines what foods are edible, or allowable, in the diet. This idea is not always based on the nutritional value, or the visual appeal. Considerations include:
  - Whether the food is perceived as harmful
  - What foods are for animal consumption (not human)
  - Whether others within the culture consume it

- The types of foods within a culture fall into three categories regarding the role they have in the diet.
  - Core foods make up the majority of dietary intake (the foods eaten most often and consistently).
  - Secondary foods are not consumed as often as core foods but are included often.
  - Peripheral foods are consumed occasionally due to cost or availability. Peripheral foods might be reserved for special days or consumed less often because they are not well-tolerated.
- Food preparation guidelines can include how the food is obtained or prepared prior to being obtained by the client, methods of cooking, and the use of seasonings.
- The timing and frequency of meals can vary across cultures.
- Foods are often linked to health beliefs, with cultures defining what foods are helpful or not, whether foods are curative, and under what conditions the foods should be consumed.
  - American culture values eating foods from food groups (fruits and vegetables, grains, proteins).
  - Many cultures (for example, Asian and Pacific Islander cultures) have health beliefs regarding hot and cold balance.
- Through acculturation, individuals and groups change their practices to reflect the dominant culture. First-generation members of a family are more likely to follow their traditional foodway, with subsequent generations incorporating the dominant culture's food practices through socialization. Acculturation of the diet can include removing or replacing traditional foods with new ones and adding new foods to the diet.
- Dietary changes resulting from acculturation can be:
  - Positive, if the client includes more healthy foods.
  - Negative, if intake of high-fat, high-calorie, or high-sodium foods increases.

SELECTED POPULATIONS

Hispanic/Latinx

This is the predominant minority group in the U.S., with the largest percentage clients being of Mexican heritage. Certain foods are considered hot or cold and can be used to provide balance for healing. Cinnamon and teas (mint, chamomile) can be used as part of healing.

NUTRITION-RELATED CONCERNS

- High intake of fruit, dark green and orange vegetables, legumes
- Increased intake of saturated fat and sodium
- Decreased intake of whole grains and milk
- High prevalence of obesity
- More than twice as likely to develop diabetes mellitus type 2

Black/African American

This is the second largest minority group in the U.S. Most individuals can identify a West African heritage or ancestors who immigrated through the Caribbean, Central America, or Eastern Africa. Food habits of black/African American clients are related more to personal factors (work schedule, location, socioeconomic status) than heritage. Black/African Americans are more likely than white Americans to accept a larger body size as normal.

NUTRITION-RELATED CONCERNS

- Score just under the national average on USDA healthy eating scores (total and saturated fat, sodium, cholesterol intake).
- Lower intake of whole grains, milk, and vegetables than clients who are white, who have a higher intake of sodium and saturated fat.
- Highest prevalence rates of obesity.
- Increased rates of diabetes mellitus with increased risk of complications.
- Increased risk for hypertension, usually uncontrolled.

Asian American/Pacific Islander

This is the third largest minority group in the U.S. and includes 37 different ethnic groups. The Chinese population is the largest subgroup of Asian American people. Common food patterns among this diverse group include devoting considerable skill and time to food preparation and consumption of rice and vegetables more than meats.

Many Asian cultures believe in the balance of yin and yang forces, and that, when food is digested, it turns into one of these components. Diseases associated with yin forces are treated by consuming yang foods, and yang illness with yin foods.

Yang foods: Fried foods, coffee, spice, meat, meat broths

Yin foods: Seaweed, many fruits and vegetables, cold beverages

NUTRITION-RELATED CONCERNS

- Lowest prevalence of obesity
- Highest life expectancy (Asian American females)
- Higher risk of diabetes mellitus type 2 when body fat increases (compared to other groups)

SELECTED CULTURAL DIETS

These diets common to the major subcultural groups in the United States can vary from client to client. Acculturation causes a moving away from the traditional foods in place of others.

American

- Many foods from various cultures are components of American cuisine.
- Foods are often prepared quickly or are expected to be made fast. Foods prepared at home often include premade ingredients or packaged kits to reduce mealtime preparation.

NUTRITIONAL HEALTH RISKS

- Convenience foods for home cooking are high in sodium and calories, while low in fiber.
- Portion sizes on packaged meal kits are often small, leading to consuming more than one serving.
- Meals and snacks eaten away from home are low in fruit, vegetables, dairy, and whole grains, but high in fat, sugar, and sodium.

Soul food

The soul food diet had its origins in Southern and Western Africa. Many Americans have adopted soul food practices, particularly in the Southern U.S. It is more common in low socioeconomic or rural areas.

TRADITIONAL FOODS: Rice, grits, cornbread, hominy, okra, greens, sweet potatoes, apples, peaches, buttermilk, pork rinds, cheddar or American cheese, ham, pork, chicken, catfish, black-eyed peas, red and pinto beans, peanuts, fruit drinks, fatback

ACCULTURATION

- Buying convenience foods rather than preparing homemade (breads, luncheon meat, cured meats)
- Increased milk consumption
- Possible reduced intake of fruits and vegetables if not readily available

NUTRITIONAL HEALTH RISKS

- High in fat, protein, and sodium
- Low in potassium, calcium, and fiber (protective nutrients)
- Many foods are fried

Mexican

Spanish and Native American cultures have influenced the traditional Mexican diet.

TRADITIONAL FOODS: Rice, corn, tortillas, tropical fruits, vegetables, nuts, legumes, eggs, cheese, seafood, poultry, infrequent sweets and red meat

- Tortillas eaten at most meals
- Animal protein from ground poultry, pork, goat
- Vegetables often incorporated into the main dish

ACCULTURATION

- Decreased intake of vegetables
- Intake of corn-based products replaced with flour-based
- Increased milk intake or replaced with low-fat options
- Red meat intake increased while legume intake decreased
- Increased use of fats (butter, margarine, salad dressing)
- Increased use of high-sugar, low-nutrient beverages (e.g., replacing fruit juice with carbonated sodas)

Chinese

Largest Asian American subgroup

TRADITIONAL FOODS: Wheat (northern), rice (southern), noodles, fruits, land and sea vegetables, nuts/seeds, soy foods (tofu), nut/seed oils, fish, shellfish, poultry, eggs, sweets, rarely red meats, seafoods, tea, beer

Tofu, soups made from bone, and fish containing small bones provide most of calcium intake.

ACCULTURATION
- Increased intake of wheat-based foods
- Increased intake of raw vegetables and replacement of traditional vegetables
- Increased fruit intake
- Increased intake of dairy, meat, ethnic dishes, and fast food

NUTRITIONAL-RELATED HEALTH RISKS
- Most foods are cooked, with exception of occasional fresh fruit.
- Risk of increased sodium is possible due to salting/drying to preserve foods and use of salt-based condiments.

Vegetarian diets

Semi-vegetarian/flexitarian diets are mainly plant-based diets with occasional intake of meat, poultry, dairy, or fish.

Vegetarian
- A vegetarian diet typically omits meat, seafood, poultry, or fish.
- Some clients include eggs, dairy products, fish, and/or occasional other animal products.

Vegan
- Pure vegan diets do not include animal products of any type, including eggs and milk products.
- A pure vegan diet requires a variety of plant materials to be consumed in specific combinations in order to ensure essential amino acid intake.
  - The vegan diet is adequate in protein with sufficient intake of nuts and legumes (dried peas, cooked beans).
  - Clients following a vegan diet should ensure adequate intake of iron, zinc, calcium, vitamin D, omega-3 fatty acids and vitamin B_{12}, because there is a risk of deficiency of these nutrients depending on the types of foods selected.
- A **raw vegan diet** is based on consuming uncooked plant-based foods.
- A **macrobiotic diet** is a whole-foods diet based on locally grown plants with occasional fish or seafood.

NUTRITIONAL-RELATED HEALTH RISKS: Risk for deficiency in vitamin B_{12}, vitamin D, iron, calcium, and zinc, unless the client incorporates these foods regularly.

6.1 Food Label Examples

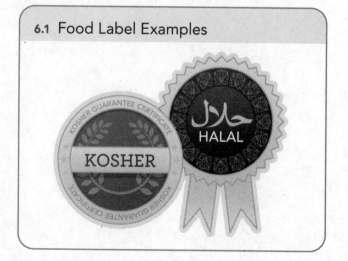

RELIGION AND NUTRITION

- Religion has a profound influence on foodways, especially because religion crosses geographic boundaries. Although culture and religion are linked, religion often has more of an influence on dietary practices than culture. Variations among individual denominations of a religion can vary greatly.
  - The dietary laws for Orthodox Judaism are outlined in the Torah.
  - Two Protestant Christian faiths prescribe dietary laws (Church of Jesus Christ of Latter-Day Saints [Mormon], Seventh Day Adventists).
  - The Qur'an contains food laws for the Islamic faith. Foods are either permitted (halal) or prohibited (haram).
  - Hindu and Buddhist religions have values related to not harming living creatures (ahimsa), which lends to followers practicing vegetarianism.
- Some followers of a particular religion follow the moral laws but not dietary prescriptions. Always ask clients to describe their dietary preferences.

Variations based on religion

Eating on Holy Days: Some religions observe feasts on specific days (Eastern Orthodox Christian, Judaism). During Passover, Judaism calls for consumption of unleavened bread only.

Fasting for religious holidays: Islam calls for fasting during Ramadan. Roman Catholicism calls for refraining from meat consumption on Ash Wednesday and Fridays during Lent, and to avoid food or beverage intake for 1 hr before communion. Seventh-Day Adventism recommends a 5- to 6-hr interval between meals. Judaism calls for a 24-hr fast during Yom Kippur.

Restricting specific substances
- Alcohol (Islam, Hindu, Mormon, Seventh-Day Adventism)
- Pork (Seventh-Day Adventism, Orthodox Judaism, Islam, Hindu, Buddhism)
- Coffee or tea (Seventh-Day Adventism, Mormonism)
- Other: Clients who follow Orthodox Judaism might not eat meat and dairy products at the same time; pareve foods contain neither and can be consumed at any time. Clients who follow Judaism might consume only fish that have scales and fins.

Consuming animal products
- Vegetarian diet: Seventh-Day Adventism, Hinduism, Buddhism
- Orthodox Judaism and Islam call for consumption of Kosher animals. Both have regulations for how animals are slaughtered, particularly so that no blood is consumed.

Preparing foods: Orthodox Judaism prohibits food preparation on the Sabbath.

NURSING INTERVENTIONS

- Obtaining the client's preferences related to nutrition is vital. The information on cultural and religious influences on nutrition is so vast that the nurse should focus more on the needs of the individual clients for whom the nurse is assigned care. Ask questions regarding the following.
  - What portions of the client's diet are influenced by personal values
  - What the client considers healthy versus unhealthy
  - What food and eating means to the client
  - When the client eats meals, and if there is a sequence to the foods eaten
  - Who shops for and prepares the foods the client consumes
  - Whether the client abstains from any foods
  - Whether there are restrictions related to foods and food preparation
  - Whether foods are linked to religious practice or spiritual beliefs
  - Whether the client's beliefs dictate fasting, feasting, or types of foods consumed on specific days or dates
- Seek further information about the client's preferred dietary practices from reputable sources, as needed, to guide nutritional counseling.
- If specific foods associated with the client's culture are deemed negative medically, ask the client to reduce consumption of the foods rather than eliminating them (reducing portion size, eating less often).
- Suggest fruits and vegetables that are similar in taste or texture to what the client prefers, to increase or ensure adequate consumption.
- Seek the assistance of a dietitian to ensure the client will receive essential nutrients and to help combine medical recommendations with personal preferences.

Active Learning Scenario

A nurse is providing teaching to a group of clients who consume a primarily Mexican diet. What cultural considerations should guide the nurse with the teaching? Use the ATI Active Learning Template: Basic Concept to complete this item to include the following.

RELATED CONTENT

- Traditional foods: Include at least six foods common to this diet.
- Acculturation: Describe three examples of how food practices change as clients who follow this diet acculturate to the dominant American culture.

Active Learning Scenario Key

Using the ATI Active Learning Template: Basic Concept

RELATED CONTENT

- Traditional foods
  - Grains: rice, corn
  - Tropical fruits and vegetables
  - Protein: nuts, legumes, eggs, cheese, seafood, poultry
- Acculturation
  - Increased milk use
  - Decreased vegetable consumption
  - Replacement of corn by wheat in tortillas and breads
  - Decreased bean use and change in rice preparation to plain boiled rice
  - Added fats in the form of butter or salad dressings on cooked vegetables and side salads
  - Replacement of fruit-based drinks by sugar-laden drinks
- Ⓝ *NCLEX® Connection: Psychosocial Integrity, Cultural Awareness/ Cultural Influences on Health*

1. A nurse is assisting a client with selecting food choices on a menu. Which of the following actions by the nurse demonstrates ethnocentrism?

   A. Asking the client about some favorite food choices

   B. Notifying the dietitian to complete the menu

   C. Recommending one's own favorite foods

   D. Asking the client's family to fill out the menu

2. A nurse is reviewing the effect of culture on nutrition during a staff in-service. Which of the following groups prescribes eating specific foods to balance forces in the body during illness? (Select all that apply.)

   A. Asian culture

   B. African culture

   C. Roman Catholicism

   D. Buddhism

3. A nurse is caring for a client who has hypertension. Which of the dietary patterns is sometimes followed by Asian clients and places clients at risk for this condition?

   A. Incorporation of plant-based foods in the diet

   B. Consumption of raw fruits

   C. Preparation of foods using sodium

   D. Focus on shellfish in the diet

4. A nurse educator is teaching a class on culture and food to a group of newly hired nurses. Which of the following statements by a nurse indicates an understanding of the teaching?

   A. "Most clients who practice Roman Catholicism do not drink caffeinated beverages."

   B. "Most clients who practice orthodox Judaism do not eat meat with dairy products."

   C. "Most clients who are Mormon eat only the protein of animals that are slaughtered under strict guidelines."

   D. "Most clients who practice Hinduism do not eat dairy products."

5. Which of these dietary laws are followed by those practicing Orthodox Judaism? (Select all that apply)

   A. Meat cannot be eaten with dairy products

   B. Pork and pork products prohibited

   C. Partial or total fasting

   D. Beef is prohibited

   E. Alcohol is prohibited

   F. Ritual slaughter of animals

6. Which of these dietary laws are followed by those practicing Islam? (Select all that apply)

   A. Meat cannot be eaten with dairy products

   B. Pork and pork products prohibited

   C. Partial or total fasting

   D. Beef is prohibited

   E. Alcohol is prohibited

   F. Ritual slaughter of animals

7. Which of these dietary laws are followed by those practicing Hinduism? (Select all that apply)

   A. Meat cannot be eaten with dairy products

   B. Pork and pork products prohibited

   C. Partial or total fasting

   D. Beef is prohibited

   E. Alcohol is prohibited

   F. Ritual slaughter of animals

Application Exercises Key

1. C. **CORRECT:** When generating solutions to assist the client with food choices, the nurse should incorporate the client's preferences and not demonstrate ethnocentrism by recommending one's own favorite foods.

   Ⓝ *NCLEX® Connection: Psychosocial Integrity, Cultural Awareness/ Cultural Influences on Health*

2. A, D. **CORRECT:** When taking actions, the nurse educator should teach the staff that Asian traditions can include balancing yin and yang forces within the body, and foods are grouped into those categories..

   Ⓝ *NCLEX® Connection: Psychosocial Integrity, Cultural Awareness/ Cultural Influences on Health*

3. C. **CORRECT:** The preparation of foods using sodium places the client at risk for hypertension. Many spices in the Asian diet contain sodium, or it is used as a preservative. The client should reduce sodium consumption. The client should reduce sodium consumption.

   Ⓝ *NCLEX® Connection: Health Promotion and Maintenance, High-Risk Behaviors*

4. B. **CORRECT:** When evaluating outcomes for teaching related to cultures and foods, the nurse educator recognizes that the statement, "Most clients who practice Orthodox Judaism do not eat meat with dairy products" indicates understanding of the teaching. Most clients who follow the teachings of Islam eat only the protein of animals that are slaughtered under strict guidelines.

   Ⓝ *NCLEX® Connection: Health Promotion and Maintenance, High-Risk Behaviors*

5. A, B, C, F. **CORRECT:** When evaluating outcomes for teaching related to cultures and foods, the nurse educator recognizes that the statement, "Most clients who practice Orthodox Judaism do not eat meat with dairy products" indicates understanding of the teaching.

   Ⓝ *NCLEX® Connection: Health Promotion and Maintenance, High-Risk Behaviors*

6. B, C, E, F. **CORRECT:** The dietary laws of prohibiting pork and pork products as well as alcohol, participating in partial or total fasting, and ritual slaughter of animals pertain to the religion of Islam.

   Ⓝ *NCLEX® Connection: Health Promotion and Maintenance, High-Risk Behaviors*

7. C, D. **CORRECT:** Dietary laws including participating in partial or total fasting and the prohibition of eating beef pertain to the religion of Hinduism.

   Ⓝ *NCLEX® Connection: Health Promotion and Maintenance, High-Risk Behaviors*

UNIT 1   PRINCIPLES OF NUTRITION

CHAPTER 7   # Nutrition Across the Lifespan

Nutritional needs change as clients pass through the stages of the lifespan, reflecting physiological changes.

Nurses must address nutritional needs across the lifespan and have a thorough understanding of how needs change. This includes planning and implementing dietary plans that meet clients' specific needs and assist in health promotion.

Major stages of the lifespan that have specific nutritional needs include pregnancy and lactation, infancy, childhood, adolescence, and adulthood and older adulthood.

General guidelines

- The Dietary Guidelines for Americans advocates healthy food selections: a variety of fiber-rich fruits and vegetables, whole grains, low-fat or fat-free milk and milk products, lean meats, poultry, fish, legumes, eggs, and nuts. Recommendations include nutrient-dense foods and beverages. The 2020-2025 Guidelines provide four overarching Guidelines to encourage healthy eating patterns for each stage of life.
- Follow a healthy dietary pattern at every stage of life
  - For about the first 6 months of life, exclusively feed infants human milk or iron-fortified infant formula if human milk is not available. Provide supplemental vitamin D beginning soon after birth.
  - At about 6 months, introduce nutrient-dense complimentary food that include a variety of foods from all food groups.
  - From 12 months through older adulthood, follow a healthy dietary pattern that meets nutrient needs, achieves a healthy body weight, and reduces the risk of developing chronic disease.
- Customize and enjoy nutrient-dense food and beverage choices to reflect personal preferences, cultural traditions, and budgetary considerations.

Pregnancy and lactation

- Prepregnancy nutrition is highly significant and plays an important role, because early fetal development occurs before a client might realize they are pregnant. A client should be well-nourished and within the normal weight range prior to conception. Low levels of folate prior to conception increases the likelihood of neural tube defects.
- Good nutrition during pregnancy is essential for the health of the unborn child.
- Maternal nutritional demands are increased for the development of the placenta, enlargement of the uterus, formation of amniotic fluid, increase in blood volume, and preparation of the breasts for lactation.
- A daily increase of 340 calories is recommended during the second trimester of pregnancy, and an increase of 452 calories is recommended during the third trimester of pregnancy.
- The nutritional requirements of clients who are pregnant or lactating involves more than increased caloric intake. Specific dietary requirements for major nutrients and micronutrients should be met.

DIETARY GUIDELINES

- Achieving an appropriate amount of weight gain during pregnancy prepares a client for the energy demands of labor and lactation and contributes to the birth of a newborn of normal birth weight.
- The recommended weight gain during pregnancy varies for each client depending on their body mass index (BMI) and weight prior to pregnancy.
- Lactating clients require an increase in daily caloric intake. If the client is breastfeeding during the postpartum period, an additional daily intake of 330 calories is recommended during the first 6 months, and an additional daily intake of 400 calories is recommended during the second 6 months.

7.1 Recommended weight gain during pregnancy

FIRST TRIMESTER: Recommended weight gain is 1.1 to 4.4 lb.

SECOND AND THIRD TRIMESTERS: Recommended weight gain is 2 to 4 lb/month.
- **Normal weight client (BMI 18.5–24.9):** 1 lb/week for a total of 25 to 35 lb.
- **Underweight client (BMI < 18.5):** just more than 1 lb/week for a total of 28 to 40 lb.
- **Overweight client (BMI 25–29.9):** 0.66 lb/week for a total of 15 to 25 lb.
- **Obese client (BMI > 30):** 0.5 lb/week for a total of 11 to 20 lb.

MAJOR AND MICRONUTRIENT REQUIREMENTS

- Dietary requirements for major nutrients
  - Protein should comprise 20% of the daily total calorie intake. The Dietary Reference Intake (DRI) for protein during pregnancy is 71 g/day. Protein is essential for rapid tissue growth of maternal and fetal structures, amniotic fluid, and extra blood volume. Clients who are pregnant should be aware that animal sources of protein might contain large amounts of fats.
  - Fat should be limited to 30% of total daily calorie intake.
  - Carbohydrates should comprise 50% of the total daily calorie intake. Ensuring adequate carbohydrate intake allows for protein to be spared and available for the synthesis of fetal tissue.
- The need for most vitamins and minerals increases during pregnancy and lactation. Vitamins are essential for blood formation, absorption of iron, and development of fetal tissue. TABLE 7.2 lists the comparative DRIs of major vitamins for clients age 19 to 30 during nonpregnancy, pregnancy, and lactation.

ADDITIONAL DIETARY RECOMMENDATIONS

Fluid: 2,000 to 3,000 mL fluids daily from food and drinks. Preferred fluids include water, fruit juice, and milk. Carbonated beverages and fruit drinks provide little or no nutrients.

Alcohol: It is recommended that clients abstain from alcohol consumption during pregnancy. There is no safe recommendation for alcohol use during pregnancy.

Caffeine: Caffeine crosses the placenta and can affect the movement and heart rate of the fetus. However, moderate use (less than 200 mg/day) does not appear to be harmful.

Vegetarian diets: Well-balanced vegetarian diets that include dairy products can provide all the nutritional requirements of pregnancy.

Folic acid intake: It is recommended that 600 mcg/day of folic acid be taken during pregnancy. Current recommendations for lactating clients include 500 mcg/day folic acid. It is necessary for the neurologic development of the fetus and to prevent birth defects. It is essential for maternal red blood cell formation. Clients who have had a child born with a neural tube defect should consume 4 mg daily of folic acid during pregnancy. Food sources include green leafy vegetables, enriched grains, and orange juice.

- Folic acid is the synthetic form of folate and is absorbed better by the body. Folic acid is found in supplements and in fortified foods.
- Folate is found in natural foods.

Iron: The DRI for iron increases by 50% during pregnancy to support the increase in maternal blood volume and to provide iron for fetal liver storage. Iron can be obtained from meats, eggs, leafy greens, enriched breads, and dried fruits. Consuming foods high in vitamin C aids in the absorption of iron. It is recommended that pregnant clients take a supplement of 27 to 30 mg iron daily to assure adequate intake.

Nonnutritive sweeteners: Several nonnutritive sweeteners have been approved for use during pregnancy. Occasional use is not considered harmful, but it is not known if they are beneficial.

Fish: The FDA has issued advisories regarding fish and shellfish consumption during pregnancy due to the risk of mercury levels. Mercury can be toxic to developing fetal brain tissue. Fish are a good source of omega 3 fatty acids, which are important for fetal brain and eye development.

- Limit albacore tuna to 6 oz/week.
- Avoid tilefish, shark, swordfish, marlin, orange roughy, and king mackerel due to mercury content.
- Limit weekly consumption of seafood to 12 oz.

DIETARY COMPLICATIONS

Nausea and constipation are common during pregnancy.

- For nausea, eat dry crackers, toast, and salty or tart foods. Avoid alcohol, caffeine, fats, and spices. Avoid drinking fluids with meals, and do not take medications to control nausea without checking with the provider.
- For constipation, increase fluid consumption (at least 8 cups per day) and include extra fiber in the diet. Fruits, vegetables, and whole grains contain fiber.
- Regular physical activity can minimize or prevent constipation.

Maternal phenylketonuria (PKU) is a maternal genetic disease in which high levels of phenylalanine pose danger to the fetus.

- It is important for a client to start the PKU diet at least 3 months prior to pregnancy, and continue the diet throughout pregnancy.
- The diet should include foods low in phenylalanine. Foods high in protein (fish, poultry, meat, eggs, nuts, dairy products) must be avoided due to high phenylalanine levels. Qs
- The client's blood phenylalanine levels should be monitored during pregnancy.
- These interventions will prevent fetal complications (intellectual disability, behavioral problems).

7.2 DRIs of major vitamins

NUTRIENT	NONPREGNANT	PREGNANT	LACTATING
Protein	46 g	71 g	71 g
Vitamin A	700 mcg	770 mcg	1,300 mcg
Vitamin C	75 mg	85 mg	120 mg
Vitamin D*	15 mcg	15 mcg	15 mcg
Vitamin E	15 mcg	15 mcg	19 mcg
Vitamin K*	90 mcg	90 mcg	90 mcg
Thiamin	1.1 mg	1.4 mg	1.4 mg
Vitamin B$_6$	1.3 mg	1.9 mg	2.0 mg
Folic acid	400 mcg	600 mcg	500 mcg
Vitamin B$_{12}$	2.4 mcg	2.6 mcg	2.8 mcg
Calcium*	1,000 mg	1,000 mg	1,000 mg
Iron	18 mg	27 mg	9 mg

*Values represent adequate intakes.

Source: Office of Dietary Supplements. National Institutes of Health, ods.od.nih.gov

ASSESSMENT/DATA COLLECTION AND INTERVENTIONS

- Nursing assessments should include a complete profile of the client's knowledge base regarding nutritional requirements during pregnancy.
- Nurses should review with the client the recommended dietary practices for pregnant and lactating clients, while providing materials containing this information.

Infancy

- Growth rate during infancy is more rapid than any other period of the life cycle. It is important to understand normal growth patterns to determine the adequacy of an infant's nutritional intake.
- Birth weight doubles by 4 to 6 months and triples by 1 year of age. The need for calories and nutrients is high to support the rapid rate of growth.
- Appropriate weight gain averages 0.11 to 0.21 kg (4 to 7 oz) per week during the first 4 to 6 months.
- An infant grows approximately 2.5 cm (1 in) per month in height during the first 6 months, and approximately 1.25 cm (0.5 in) per month during the second 6 months.
- Head circumference increases rapidly during the first 6 months at a rate of 1.5 cm (0.6 in) per month. The rate slows to 0.5 cm/month for months 6 to 12. By 1 year, head size should have increased by 33%. This is reflective of the growth of the nervous system.
  - The American Academy of Pediatrics (AAP) recommends the exclusive breastfeeding for infants for at least the first 6 months of age and up to 2 years of age or longer if desired. Iron-fortified infant formula is an alternative if human milk is not available. Infants can receive vitamin D supplements following birth if consuming less than 28 ounces of human milk or formula.
  - At about 6 months, introduce nutrient-dense complementary foods that include a variety of foods from all food groups along with human milk or formula.
  - From 12 months through older adulthood, follow a healthy dietary pattern that meets nutrient needs, achieves a healthy body weight, and reduces the risk of developing chronic disease.
- Semisolid foods should not be introduced before 6 months of age to coincide with the development of the gastrointestinal system, head control, ability to sit, and the back-and-forth motion of the tongue.
- Gestational iron stores begin to deplete around 4 months of age, so iron supplementation could be prescribed for infants if indicated. Once solid foods are introduced, iron-fortified cereal is a good source of iron.
- Cow's milk should not be introduced into the diet until after 1 year of age because protein and mineral content stress the immature kidney. A young infant cannot fully digest the protein and fat contained in cow's milk.

MEETING NUTRITIONAL NEEDS

Additional information about feeding is available in the Maternal Newborn Review Module (Newborn Nutrition chapter) and the Pediatric Nursing Review Module (Health Promotion of Infants chapter).

BREASTFEEDING

- A goal of Healthy People 2030 is to increase the proportion of infants who are 6 months and 12 months of age to exclusive breastfeeding.
- The Centers for Disease Control and Prevention (CDC), World Health Organization (WHO), and the American Academy of Pediatrics (AAP) recommend that infants receive breast milk solely until 6 months of age and breastfeeding should be continued while introducing complementary foods up to 2 years of age, or longer.
- Donor milk can be considered in certain circumstances.
  - The choice to feed an infant human milk from a source other than the infant's parent should be made in consultation with the provider, because the nutritional needs of each infant depend on many factors, including the infant's age and health.
  - The FDA recommends that if an infant is to be fed human milk from a source other than the infant's parent, use only milk from a source that has screened its donors and take other precautions to ensure the safety of the milk. Qs
- The AAP recommends that for the first 6 months, infants should receive no water or formula except in cases of medical indication or informed parental choice. In the hospital, no water or formula should be given to a breastfed infant unless prescribed by a provider. QEBP

Nutritional advantages of breast milk

- Carbohydrates, proteins, and fats in breast milk are predigested for ready absorption.
- Breast milk is high in omega-3 fatty acids.
- Breast milk is low in sodium.
- Iron, zinc, and magnesium found in breast milk are highly absorbable.
- Calcium absorption is enhanced, as the calcium-to-phosphorous ratio is 2:1.

Breastfeeding teaching points

- The newborn is offered the breast immediately after birth and frequently thereafter. There should be eight to 12 feedings in a 24-hr period.
- Instruct the client to demand-feed the infant and to assess for hunger cues. These include rooting, suckling on hands and fingers, and rapid eye movement. Crying is a late indicator of hunger.
- The newborn should nurse up to 15 min per breast. Findings that indicate the newborn has completed the feeding include the slowing of newborn suckling, a softened breast, or sleeping. Eventually, the infant will empty a breast within 5 to 10 min, but might need to continue to suck to meet comfort needs. QEBP
- Do not offer the newborn any supplements unless indicated by the provider.
- Frequent feedings (every 2 hr can be indicated) and manual expression of milk to initiate flow can be needed.
- Awaken the infant to feed every 3 hr during the day and every 4 hr at night.
- Encourage clients to express breast milk for supplementation if extra fluids or calories are required.

- Expressed milk can be refrigerated in sterile bottles or storage bags and labeled with the date and time the milk was expressed. It can be maintained in the refrigerator for 4 days or frozen in sterile containers for 6 months.
- Thaw milk in the refrigerator. It can be stored for 24 hr after thawing. Defrosting or heating in a microwave oven is not recommended because high heat destroys some of milk's antibodies, and can burn the infant's oral mucosa.
- Do not refreeze thawed milk.
- Unused breast milk must be discarded.
- Limit alcohol and caffeine while breastfeeding.
- Begin manual expression of the breast or use an electric breast pump if the infant is unable to breastfeed due to prematurity or respiratory distress.

FORMULA FEEDING

Can be used in place of breastfeeding, as an occasional supplement to breastfeeding, or when exclusively breastfed infants are weaned before 12 months of age.

- Commercial infant formulas provide an alternative to breast milk. They are modified from cow's milk to provide comparable nutrients. However, breast milk is superior to any formula and even more crucial for a premature infant.
- If formula-fed, an iron-fortified formula is recommended for at least the first 12 months of life or until the infant consumes adequate solid food.
- Fluoride supplements can be required if an adequate level is not supplied by the water supply.
- Precisely follow the manufacturer's mixing directions.
- Bottles of mixed formula or open cans of liquid formula require refrigeration. Do not use if the formula has been left at room temperature for 2 hr or longer. Do not reuse partially emptied bottles of formula.
- Formula can be fed chilled, warmed, or at room temperature. Always give formula at approximately the same temperature.
- The infant should not drink more than 32 oz formula per 24 hr period unless directed by a provider.

BOTTLE FEEDING

- Hold the infant during feedings with the head slightly elevated to facilitate passage of formula or breast milk into the stomach. Tilt the bottle to maintain liquid in the nipple and prevent the swallowing of air.
- Do not prop the bottle or put an infant to bed with a bottle. This practice promotes tooth decay.

INTRODUCING SOLID FOOD

- Indicators for readiness include voluntary control of the head and trunk, sit up alone or with minimal support, opens mouth when food is offered, opens mouth when food is offered, and brings items to their mouth.
- Solid food choices may be introduced in any order. Introduce one single-ingredient new food from any food group every 3 to 5 days and monitor for allergy or intolerance, which can include fussiness, rash, upper respiratory distress, vomiting, diarrhea, or constipation. Q EBP
- The infant can be ready for three meals per day with three snacks by 8 months of age.
- Homemade baby food is an acceptable feeding option. Do not use canned or packaged foods that are high in sodium. Select fresh or frozen foods, and do not add sugars or other seasonings.
- Open jars of infant food can be stored in the refrigerator for up to 24 hr.
- By 9 months of age, the infant should be able to eat table foods that are cooked, chopped, and unseasoned.
- Do not feed the infant honey due to the risk of botulism.
- Appropriate finger foods include ripe bananas, toast strips, graham crackers, cheese cubes, noodles, and peeled chunks of apples, pears, or peaches.
- Avoid giving infant, who is less than 12 months of age, foods that are considered risk for choking hazard: grapes, nuts, raw carrots.

NUTRITION-RELATED PROBLEMS

Colic

Colic is characterized by persistent crying lasting 3 hr or longer per day.
- The cause of colic is unknown, but usually occurs in the late afternoon, more than 3 days per week for more than 3 weeks. The crying is accompanied by a tense abdomen and legs drawn up to the belly.
- If breastfeeding, eliminate cruciferous vegetables (cauliflower, broccoli, and Brussels sprouts), cow's milk, onion, and chocolate, and limit caffeine and nicotine.
- Burp the infant in an upright position.

Lactose intolerance

Lactose intolerance is the inability to digest significant amounts of lactose (the predominant sugar of milk) and is due to inadequate lactase (the enzyme that digests lactose into glucose and galactose).
- Lactose intolerance has an increased prevalence in individuals of Asian, Native American, African, Latino, and Mediterranean descent.
- Findings include abdominal distention, flatus, and occasional diarrhea.
- Soy-based or casein hydrolysate formulas can be prescribed as alternative formulas for infants who are lactose intolerant.

Failure to thrive

Failure to thrive is defined as inadequate gains in weight and height in comparison to established growth and development norms (weight-for-length less than 5th percentile or weight for age below the 3rd percentile).

- Assess for findings of congenital defects, central nervous system disorders, or partial intestinal obstruction.
- Monitor for swallowing or sucking problems.
- Identify feeding patterns, especially concerning preparation of formulas.
- Observe for psychosocial problems, especially impaired caregiver-infant bonding, abuse/neglect.
- Provide supportive nutritional guidance. Usually a high-calorie, high-protein diet is indicated.
- Provide supportive parenting guidance.

Diarrhea

Diarrhea is characterized by the passage of more than three loose, watery stools over a 24-hr period.

- Overfeeding and food intolerances are common causes of osmotic diarrhea.
- Infectious diarrhea in the infant is commonly caused by rotavirus.
- Mild diarrhea can require no specific interventions. Check with the provider for any diet modifications.
- Treatment for moderate diarrhea should begin at home with oral rehydration solutions. After each loose stool, an 8 oz solution should be given. Sports drinks are contraindicated.
- Educate parents about the findings of dehydration: listlessness, sunken eyes, sunken fontanels, decreased tears, dry mucous membranes, and decreased urine output.
- Breastfed infants should continue nursing.
- Formula-fed infants usually do not require diluted formulas or special formulas.
- Contact the provider if findings of dehydration are present, or if vomiting, bloody stools, high fever, change in mental status, or refusal to take liquids occurs.

Constipation

Constipation is the inability or difficulty to evacuate the bowels.

- Constipation is not a common problem for breastfed infants.
- Constipation can be caused by formula that is too concentrated.
- Stress the importance of accurate dilution of formula.
- Advise adherence to the recommended amount of formula intake for age.

NURSING ASSESSMENT/DATA COLLECTION INTERVENTIONS

- Nursing assessments should include an assessment of knowledge base of the client regarding nutritional guidelines for infants, normal infant growth patterns, breastfeeding, formula feeding, and the progression for the introduction of solid foods.
- Additionally, nurses should provide education and references for the client regarding each of the assessments listed above.

Childhood

- Growth rate slows following infancy.
- MyPlate.gov is a food guidance system that offers an Internet-based tool to provide clients with individualized recommendations for adequate nutrition. Children require the same food groups as adults, but in smaller serving sizes. Qι
- Energy needs and appetite vary with the child's activity level and growth rate.
- Generally, nutrient needs increase with age.
- Attitudes toward food and general food habits are established by 5 years of age.
- Increasing the variety and texture of foods helps the child develop good eating habits.
- Foods like hot dogs, popcorn, peanuts, grapes, raw carrots, celery, peanut butter, tough meat, and candy can cause choking or aspiration. Qs
- Inclusion in family mealtime is important for social development.
- Group eating becomes a significant means of socialization for school-age children.

TODDLERS: 1 TO 3 YEARS OLD

NUTRITION GUIDELINES

- Toddlers generally grow 2 to 3 inches in height and gain approximately 5 to 6 lb/year.
- Limit 100% juice to 4 to 6 oz a day.
- The 1- to 2-year-old child requires whole cow's milk to provide adequate fat for the still-growing brain.
- Food serving size is 1 tbsp for each year of age.
- Exposure to a new food might be needed 15 to 20 times before the child develops an acceptance of it.
- If there is a negative family history for allergies, cow's milk, chocolate, citrus fruits, egg white, seafood, and nut butters can be gradually introduced while monitoring the child for reactions.
- Toddlers prefer finger foods because of their increasing autonomy. They prefer plain foods to mixtures, but usually like macaroni and cheese, spaghetti, and pizza.
- Regular meal times and nutritious snacks best meet nutrient needs.
- Snacks or desserts that are high in sugar, fat, or sodium should be avoided.
- Children are at an increased risk for choking until 4 years of age.
- Avoid foods that are potential choking hazards. Always provide adult supervision during snack and mealtimes. During food preparation, cut small, bite-sized pieces that are easy to swallow to prevent choking. Do not allow the child to engage in drinking or eating during play activities or while lying down. Qs

NUTRITIONAL CONCERN/RISKS

Iron

- Iron deficiency anemia is the most common nutritional deficiency disorder in children.
- Lean red meats provide sources of readily absorbable iron.
- Consuming vitamin C (orange juice, tomatoes) with plant sources of iron (beans, raisins, peanut butter, whole grains) will maximize absorption.
- Milk should be limited to the recommended quantities (24 oz) because it is a poor source of iron and can displace the intake of iron-rich foods.

Vitamin D

- Vitamin D is essential for bone development.
- Recommended vitamin D intake is the same (5 mcg/day) from birth through age 50. Children require more vitamin D because their bones are growing.
- Milk (cow, soy) and fatty fish are good sources of vitamin D.
- Sunlight exposure leads to vitamin D synthesis. Children who spend large amounts of time inside (watching TV, playing video games) are at an increased risk for vitamin D deficiency.
- Vitamin D assists in the absorption of calcium into the bones.

PRESCHOOLERS: 3 TO 6 YEARS

NUTRITION GUIDELINES

- Preschoolers generally grow 2 to 3 inches in height and gain approximately 5 to 6 lb/year.
- Preschoolers need to consume 13 to 19 g/day of complete protein.
- If the preschooler consumes foods from all five food groups and height and weight are within expected reference ranges, supplemental vitamins/minerals might not be needed.
- Preschoolers tend to dislike strong-tasting vegetables (cabbage, onions), but like many raw vegetables that are eaten as finger foods.
- Food jags (ritualistic preference for one food) are common and usually short-lived.
- MyPlate guidelines are appropriate, requiring the lowest number of servings per food group.
- Food patterns and preferences are first learned from the family, and peers begin influencing preferences and habits at around 5 years of age.

NUTRITIONAL CONCERNS/RISKS

Concerns include overfeeding; intake of high-calorie, high-fat, high-sodium snacks, soft drinks, and juices; and inadequate intake of fruits and vegetables.
- Be alert to the appropriate serving size of foods (1 tbsp per year of age).
- Avoid high-fat and high-sugar snacks.
- Encourage daily physical activities.
- Can switch to skim or 1% low-fat milk after 2 years of age.

Iron deficiency anemia

Lead poisoning is a risk for children younger than 6 years of age because they frequently place objects in their mouths that can contain lead and have a higher rate of intestinal absorption.
- Feed children at frequent intervals because more lead is absorbed on an empty stomach. **Qs**
- Inadequate intake of calories, calcium, iron, zinc, and phosphorous can increase susceptibility.

SCHOOL-AGE CHILDREN: 6 TO 12 YEARS

NUTRITION GUIDELINES

- School-age children generally grow 2 to 3 inches in height and gain approximately 5 to 6 lb/year.
- Following MyPlate recommendations, the diet should provide variety, balance, and moderation.
- Young athletes need to meet energy, protein, and fluid needs.
- Educate children to make healthy food selections.
- Children enjoy learning how to safely prepare nutritious snacks.
- Children need to learn to eat snacks only when hungry, not when bored or inactive.

NUTRITIONAL CONCERNS/RISKS

Not eating breakfast occurs in about 10% of children.
- Optimum performance in school is dependent on a nutritious breakfast.
- Children who regularly eat breakfast tend to have an age-appropriate BMI.

Overweight/obesity affects about 41% of children.
- Greater psychosocial implications exist for children than adults.
- Overweight children tend to be obese adults.
- Prevention is essential. Encourage healthy eating habits, decrease fats and sugars (empty-calorie foods), and increase the level of physical activity.
- A weight-loss program directed by a provider is indicated for children who are overweight, or obese if they have comorbidity. Otherwise, efforts are directed at maintaining weight so the BMI will normalize as height increases.
- Praise the child's abilities and skills.
- Never use food as a reward or punishment.

NURSING ASSESSMENT/DATA COLLECTION AND INTERVENTIONS

Nursing assessments should include the parent's knowledge base of the child's nutritional requirements, and nutritional concerns with regard to age. Nurses should provide education for the parent and child about nutritional recommendations.

Adolescence

- The rate of growth during adolescence is second only to the rate in infancy. Nutritional needs for energy, protein, calcium, iron, and zinc increase at the onset of puberty and the growth spurt.
- The female adolescent growth spurt usually begins at 10 or 11 years of age, peaks at 12 years, and is completed by 17 years. Female energy requirements are less than that of males, as they experience less growth of muscle and bone tissue and more fat deposition.
- The male adolescent growth spurt begins at 12 or 13 years of age, peaks at 14 years, and is completed by 21 years.
- Eating habits of adolescents are often inadequate in meeting recommended nutritional intake goals.

NUTRITIONAL CONSIDERATIONS

- Energy requirements average 2,000 cal/day for a 12- to 18-year-old female and 2,200 to 2,800 cal/day for a 12- to 18-year-old male.
- The USDA reports that the average U.S. adolescent consumes a diet deficient in folate, vitamins A and E, iron, zinc, magnesium, calcium, and fiber. This trend is more pronounced in females than males.
- Diets of adolescents generally exceed recommendations for total fat, saturated fat, cholesterol, sodium, and sugar.

NUTRITIONAL RISKS

Eating and snacking patterns promote essential nutrient deficiencies (calcium, vitamins, iron, fiber) and overconsumption of sugars, fat, and sodium.

- Adolescents tend to skip meals, especially breakfast, and eat more meals away from home.
- Foods are often selected from vending machines, convenience stores, and fast food restaurants. These foods are typically high in fat, sugar, and sodium.
- Carbonated beverages can replace milk and fruit juices in the diet with resulting deficiencies in vitamin C, riboflavin, phosphorous, and calcium.

Increased need for iron

- Females 14 to 18 years of age require 15 mg/day of iron to support expansion of blood volume and blood loss during menstruation.
- Males 14 to 18 years of age require 11 mg/day of iron to support expansion of muscle mass and blood volume.

Inadequate calcium intake can predispose the adolescent to osteoporosis later in life.

- During adolescence, 45% of bone mass is added.
- Normal blood-calcium levels are maintained by drawing calcium from the bones if calcium intake is low.
- Adolescents require at least 1,300 mg/day of calcium, which can be achieved by three to four servings from the dairy food group.

Dieting

- The stigma of obesity and social pressure to be thin can lead to unhealthy eating practices and poor body image, especially in females.
- Males are more susceptible to using supplements and high-protein drinks in order to build muscle mass and improve athletic performance. Some athletes restrict calories to maintain or achieve a lower weight.
- Eating disorders can follow self-imposed crash diets for weight loss.

Eating disorders (anorexia nervosa, bulimia nervosa, binge eating disorder) commonly begin during adolescence. These disorders are discussed further in the **MENTAL HEALTH REVIEW MODULE, CHAPTER 19: EATING DISORDERS.**

Adolescent pregnancy

- The physiologic demands of a growing fetus compromise the adolescent's needs for their own unfinished growth and development.
- Inconsistent eating and poor food choices place the adolescent at risk for anemia, pregnancy-induced hypertension, gestational diabetes, premature labor, miscarriage, and birth of a newborn of low birth weight.

NURSING ASSESSMENT/DATA COLLECTION AND INTERVENTIONS

- Nursing assessments should include a determination of the following in the adolescent.
  - Typical 24-hr food intake
  - Weight patterns, current weight, and body mass index (BMI)
  - Attitude about current weight
  - Use of nutritional supplements, vitamins, and minerals
  - Medical history and use of prescription medications
  - Use of over-the-counter medications
  - Use of substances (marijuana, alcohol, tobacco)
  - Level of daily physical activity
- Assess for findings of an eating disorder. This can include an evaluation of the adolescent's laboratory values.
- Nursing assessments should include strategies that promote health for the adolescent.
  - Educate the adolescent on using MyPlate to meet energy and nutrient needs with three regular meals and snacks.
  - Stress the importance of meeting calcium needs by including low-fat milk, yogurt, and cheese in the diet.

- Educate the adolescent on how to select and prepare nutrient-dense snack foods: unbuttered, unsalted popcorn; pretzels; fresh fruit; string cheese; smoothies made with low-fat yogurt, skim milk, or reduced-calorie fruit juice; and raw vegetables with low-fat dips. Qᴘᴄᴄ
- Encourage participation in vigorous physical activity at least three times per week.
- Refer pregnant adolescents to the Women, Infant, and Children (WIC) nutrition subsidy program.
- Provide individual and group counseling for adolescents who have findings of eating disorders.

Adulthood and older adulthood

The 2020-2025 Guidelines provide four overarching guidelines to encourage healthy eating patterns for each stage of life.

- Follow a healthy dietary pattern at every stage of life
- Customize and enjoy nutrient-dense food and beverage choices to reflect personal preferences, cultural traditions, and budgetary considerations.
  - The Dietary Guidelines provide a framework that is designed for customization for individual needs and preferences as well as foodways of diverse cultures.
- Focus on meeting food group needs with nutrient-dense foods and beverages and stay within calorie limits.
  - Core elements of a healthy dietary pattern include:
    - Vegetables of all types (dark green; red and orange; beans, peas, and lentils; starchy; and other vegetables
    - Fruits (especially whole fruits)
    - Grains (at least half should be whole grain)
    - Dairy (fat-free or low-fat milk, yogurt and cheese or alternatives if needed)
    - Protein foods (lean meats, poultry, and eggs; seafood; beans, peas, and lentils' nuts, seeds, and soy products)
    - Oils (vegetable oils and oils in foods such as seafood and nuts)
- Limit foods and beverages higher in added sugars, saturated fat, and sodium, and limit alcoholic beverage.
  - Foods and beverages high in added sugars, saturated fat, or sodium as well as alcoholic beverages should be limited.
    - Added sugars: Less than 10% of cal/day starting at age 2 and avoid foods and beverages with added sugars for those younger than age 2
    - Saturated fat: Choose monounsaturated and polyunsaturated fats from fish, lean meats, nuts, and vegetable oils. Less than 10% of cal/day starting at age 2.
    - Sodium: Consume less than 2,300 mg/day (about 1 tsp) of salt by limiting most canned and processed foods. Prepare foods without adding salt.
    - Alcoholic beverages: Drinking less is better for health. If choosing to drink alcohol, drink in moderation by limiting intake to 2 drinks of less/day for men and 1 drink or less in a day for women.

- A balanced diet for all adults consists of 45% to 65% carbohydrates and 20% to 35% fat (with 10% or less from saturated fats).
- The recommended amount for protein is unchanged in adults and older adults. However, many nutrition experts believe that protein requirements increase in older adults.
- Older adults need to reduce total caloric intake. This is due to the decrease in basal metabolic rate that occurs from the decrease in lean body mass that develops with aging.
- Reduced caloric intake predisposes the older adult for development of nutrient deficiencies.
- Older adults can have physical, mental, and social changes that affect their ability to purchase, prepare, and digest foods and nutrients.
- Dehydration is the most common fluid and electrolyte imbalance in older adults. Fluid needs increase with medication-induced fluid losses. Some disease processes necessitate fluid restrictions.
- BMI should be between 18.5 and 24.9. There is an increased risk for both overweight and underweight older adult clients. Overweight adults are more prone to hypertension, diabetes mellitus, and stroke.

NUTRITIONAL CONCERNS

- A 24-hr dietary intake is helpful in determining the need for dietary education.
- Older adults can have oral problems (ill-fitting dentures, difficulty chewing or swallowing), and a decrease in salivation or poor dental health.
- Older adults have decreased cellular function and reduced body reserves, leading to decreased absorption of multiple vitamins and minerals as well as reductions in insulin production and sensitivity.
- Older adults have a decreased lean muscle mass. Exercise can help to counteract muscle mass loss.
- The loss of calcium can result in decreased bone density in older adults.

BALANCED DIET AND NUTRIENT NEEDS

MyPlate suggests the following daily food intake for adults and older adults who get less than 30 min of moderate physical activity most days.

Grains: Select whole grains.

Vegetables: Select orange and dark green leafy vegetables.

Fruits: Select fresh, dried, canned, or juices. Avoid fruits with added sugar. Make half your plate vegetables and fruits.

Milk, yogurt, and cheese group: One cup of milk or plain yogurt is equivalent to 1 1/2 oz natural cheese or 2 oz processed cheese.

Protein foods group: Includes meat, fish, poultry, dry beans, eggs, soy products, seeds, and nuts. One ounce-equivalent equals 1 oz meat, fish, or poultry (baked, grilled, broiled); 1/4; cup cooked beans; 1 egg; 1 tbsp peanut butter; or 1/2; oz nuts or seeds. Use lean meats.

Oils: Use vegetable oils (except palm and coconut). One tbsp of oil equals 3 tsp equivalent; 1 tbsp equals 2 1/2; tsp dietary intake; and 1 oz nuts equals 3 tsp oils (except hazelnut, which equals 4 tsp).

Discretionary calories: 132 to 362 discretionary calories are permitted per day. These add up quickly and can be from more than one food group.

Minerals: Calcium requirements increase for older adults as the efficiency of calcium absorption decreases with age.

Vitamins: Vitamins A, D, C, E, B_6, and B_{12} can be decreased in older adults. Supplemental vitamins are recommended.

REGULAR EXERCISE

- All adults should exercise at a moderate or vigorous pace for at least 150 min per week. Adults who cannot do 150 min of moderate activity should be as physically active as tolerated.
- Moderate activities include gardening/yard work, golf, dancing, and walking briskly.
- The loss of lean muscle mass is part of normal aging and can be decreased with regular exercise. The loss of lean muscle can be associated with a decrease in total protein and insulin sensitivity.
- Regular exercise can improve bone density, relieve depression, and enhance cardiovascular and respiratory function.

POTENTIAL EFFECT OF PHYSICAL, MENTAL, AND SOCIAL CHANGES

- Diseases and treatments can interfere with nutrient and food absorption, and utilization.
  - Aging adults are at an increased risk for developing osteoporosis (decreasing total bone mass and deterioration of bone tissue). Adequate calcium and vitamin D intake with regular weight-bearing exercise is important for maximizing bone density.
  - Musculoskeletal concerns, such as arthritis, cause pain that can interfere with the purchase and preparation of foods.
  - Dementia can make shopping, storing, and cooking food difficult.
- Medications can cause electrolyte losses.
- Loss of smell and vision interfere with the interest in eating food.
- Older adults can have difficulty chewing, in which case mincing or chopping food is helpful. They can have difficulty swallowing food, and thickened liquids can decrease the risk for aspiration.
- Social isolation, loss of a partner, and mental deterioration can cause poor nutrition in adult and older adult clients. Encourage socialization and refer to a senior center or program. ○PCC
- A fixed income can make it difficult for older adults to purchase needed foods. Refer to food programs, senior centers, and food banks. Meals on Wheels programs are available for housebound older adults.

FLUID INTAKE

- The long-held standard of consuming eight 8-oz glasses of liquid per day has been tempered by evidence that dehydration is not imminent even when less than 64 oz of fluid is consumed.
- Solid foods provide varying amounts of water, making it possible to get adequate fluid despite low beverage intake.
- For healthy adults, it is generally acceptable to allow normal drinking and eating habits to provide needed fluids.
- Encourage water and natural juices, and discourage drinking only soda pop and other liquids that have caffeine.

NURSING ASSESSMENT/DATA COLLECTION AND INTERVENTIONS

- Nursing assessments should include a dietary profile of the adult or older adult. Medical history, medication regimen, mobility, social practices, mental status, and financial circumstances are important components of the assessment.
- Nurses should provide education about dietary practices for the adult and older adult, while additionally providing referrals to registered dietitians and community agencies when needed

Active Learning Scenario

A community health nurse is teaching a group of guardians the importance of adequate vitamin D intake for children. Use the ATI Active Learning Template: Basic Concept to complete this item.

UNDERLYING PRINCIPLES

- Explain why vitamin D is important for children.
- Identify at least two sources of vitamin D.

Active Learning Scenario Key

Using the ATI Active Learning Template: Basic Concept
UNDERLYING PRINCIPLES
- Vitamin D is essential for the development of healthy bones. It is important in children because their bones are newly formed and continually growing.
- Vitamin D aids in the absorption of calcium into the bones. Sunlight exposure, milk (cow's, soy), and fatty fish are sources of vitamin D.
- Ⓝ *NCLEX® Connection: Health Promotion and Maintenance, Aging Process*

1. **A, B, D. CORRECT:** When taking actions, the nurse should instruct the clients who are pregnant about iron-rich foods which include beans, fish, and lean red meats. Dairy products and apples are not foods rich in iron.

Ⓝ *NCLEX® Connection: Health Promotion and Maintenance, Ante-/Intra-/Postpartum and Newborn Care*

2. **A, B, E. CORRECT:** When taking actions, the nurse should instruct the parents of a toddler that graham crackers, apple slices, and cheese cubes are appropriate snacks. Raisins and jellybeans are not appropriate snack selections because they pose a choking risk and are difficult to chew.

Ⓝ *NCLEX® Connection: Health Promotion and Maintenance, Aging Process*

3. **A, B, D. CORRECT:** When recognizing cues, the nurse should expect an infant who is lactose intolerant to have abdominal distention, flatus, and occasional diarrhea. Hypoactive bowel sounds and visible peristalsis are not associated with lactose intolerance.

Ⓝ *NCLEX® Connection: Health Promotion and Maintenance, Aging Process*

4. **A, B, C. CORRECT:** When taking actions, the school nurse should discuss healthy snack food choices with a group of adolescents, including carrot sticks with low-fat ranch dip, cheese and crackers, and unbuttered popcorn. French fries and hot dogs are not healthy food choices because they are high in fat and sodium

Ⓝ *NCLEX® Connection: Health Promotion and Maintenance, Aging Process*

5. **B, C, D. CORRECT:** When taking actions, the nurse should include the following information in nutritional education for a group of older adult clients: Age-related changes can reduce the body's ability to absorb vitamins and minerals. Adult clients should obtain 20% to 35% of daily calories from fat. Adult clients should obtain 45% to 65% of daily calories from carbohydrates. Fruits and vegetables should make up one-half of each meal. Also, protein requirement do not increase during older adulthood..

Ⓝ *NCLEX® Connection: Health Promotion and Maintenance, Health Promotion/Disease Prevention*

1. A nurse is teaching a group of clients who are pregnant about iron-rich foods. Which of the following foods should the nurse include? (Select all that apply.)
   A. Beans
   B. Fish
   C. Dairy products
   D. Lean red meats
   E. Apples

2. A nurse is educating the parents of a toddler about appropriate snack foods. Which of the following foods should the nurse include? (Select all that apply.)
   A. Graham crackers
   B. Apple slices
   C. Raisins
   D. Jelly beans
   E. Cheese cubes

3. A nurse is assessing a 6-month-old infant who has a lactose intolerance. Which of the following findings should the nurse expect? (Select all that apply.)
   A. Abdominal distention
   B. Flatus
   C. Hypoactive bowel sounds
   D. Occasional diarrhea
   E. Visible peristalsis

4. A school nurse is teaching a group of adolescents about healthy snack food choices. Which of the following foods should the nurse include? (Select all that apply.)
   A. Carrot sticks with low-fat dip
   B. Cheese and crackers
   C. Unbuttered popcorn
   D. French fries
   E. Hot dog

5. A nurse at a community center is providing nutrition counseling for a group of older adult clients. Which of the following information should the nurse include? (Select all that apply.)
   A. Increase protein to 50% of daily calories.
   B. The need for vitamins and minerals can increase.
   C. Up to 35% of daily calories should come from fat.
   D. At least 45% of daily calories should come from carbohydrates.
   E. Fruits and vegetables should make up one-third of each meal.

NCLEX® Connections

When reviewing the following chapters, keep in mind the relevant topics and tasks of the NCLEX outline, in particular:

Basic Care and Comfort

NUTRITION AND ORAL HYDRATION
Monitor the client's nutritional status. Provide client nutrition through tube feedings.

Evaluate side effects of client tube feedings and intervene as needed.

Monitor client hydration status.

Pharmacological and Parenteral Therapies

TOTAL PARENTERAL NUTRITION
Administer parenteral nutrition, and evaluate client response.

Apply knowledge of nursing procedures and psychomotor skills when caring for a client receiving TPN.

Reduction of Risk Potential

LABORATORY VALUES: Compare client laboratory values to normal laboratory values.

POTENTIAL FOR ALTERATIONS IN BODY SYSTEMS
Identify client potential for skin breakdown.

Identify client potential for aspiration.

CHAPTER 8 *Modified Diets*

Therapeutic nutrition is the role of food and nutrition in the treatment of diseases and disorders. The basic diet becomes therapeutic when modifications are made to meet client needs. Modifications can include increasing or decreasing caloric intake, fiber, or other specific nutrients; omitting specific foods; and modifying the consistency of foods.

It is important to remember, however, that food meets both physiological and psychological needs and should be a pleasant experience for the hospitalized client. Nurses should collaborate with the dietitian for nutritional or dietary concerns. Qᴛᴄ

TYPES OF MODIFIED DIETS

Regular diet (normal or house diet)

- Indicated for clients who do not need dietary restrictions. The diet is adjusted to meet age specific needs throughout the life cycle.
- Many health care facilities offer self-select menus for regular diets.
- Modify the regular diet to accommodate individual preferences, food habits, and ethnic values. Qᴘᴄᴄ

Clear liquid diet

- Consists of foods or fluids that have no residue and are liquid at room temperature.
- Primarily to prevent dehydration and relieve thirst, the diet consists of water and carbohydrates. This diet requires minimal digestion, leaves minimal residue, and is non-gas-forming. It is nutritionally inadequate and should not be used long-term.
- Indications include acute illness, reduction of colon fecal material prior to certain diagnostic tests and procedures, acute gastrointestinal disorders, and some postoperative recovery.
- Acceptable foods are water, tea, coffee, fat-free broth, carbonated beverages, clear juices, ginger ale, and gelatin.

Full liquid diet

- Consists of foods that are liquid at room temperature including plain ice cream and strained cereals. Some facilities include pureed vegetables.
- Offers more variety and nutritional support than a clear liquid diet but might require supplementation of protein and calories if used more than 3 days.
- Indications include a transition from liquid to soft diets, postoperative recovery, acute gastritis, febrile conditions, and intolerance of solid foods.
- Use cautiously with clients who have dysphagia (difficulty swallowing) unless liquids are thickened appropriately. Qs
- Many dietary manuals have removed the full liquid diet, so it might be used infrequently.

Blenderized liquid (pureed) diet

- Consists of liquids and foods that are pureed to liquid form.
- The composition and consistency of a pureed diet varies, depending on the client's needs.
- Modify with regard to calories, protein, fat, or other nutrients based on the dietary needs of the client. Qᴘᴄᴄ
- Adding broth, milk, gravy, cream, soup, tomato sauce, or fruit juice to foods in place of water provides additional calories and nutritional value.
- Each food is pureed separately to preserve individual flavor.
- Indications include clients who have chewing or swallowing difficulties, oral or facial surgery, and wired jaws.

Soft (bland, low-fiber) diet

- Contains whole foods that are low in fiber, lightly seasoned, and easily digested.
- Food supplements or snacks in between meals add calories.
- Food selections vary and can include smooth, creamy, or crisp textures. Raw fruits and vegetables, coarse breads and cereals, beans, and other potentially gas-forming foods are excluded.
- Indications include clients transitioning between full liquid and regular diets, and those who have acute infections, chewing difficulties, or gastrointestinal disorders.
- Predisposes clients to constipation.

Mechanical soft diet

- A regular diet that is modified in texture. The diet composition is altered for specific nutrient needs.
- Includes foods that require minimal chewing before swallowing (ground meats, canned fruits, softly cooked vegetables).
- Butter, gravies, sugar, or honey can be added to increase calorie intake.
- Excludes harder foods (dried fruits, most raw fruits and vegetables, foods containing seeds and nuts).
- Indications include limited chewing ability; dysphagia, poorly fitting dentures, and clients who are edentulous (without teeth); surgery to the head, neck, or mouth; and strictures of the intestinal tract.

Dysphagia diet

- Prescribed when swallowing is impaired (following a stroke).
- Manifestations of dysphagia are drooling, pocketing food, choking, or gagging.

International Dysphagia Diet: (www.iddsi.org)

LEVELS OF LIQUID CONSISTENCIES

- **Level 0 (Thin)**: Liquid that flows like water, can be consumed through cup or a straw as age appropriate.
- **Level 1 (Slightly thick)**: Liquids that are thin enough to sip through a straw but thicker than water.
- **Level 2 (Mildly thick)**: Liquids that do not maintain their shape when poured but are thickened. They can be eaten with a spoon but require considerable effort to be sipped through a straw.
- **Level 3 (Moderately thick)**: Liquids with smooth texture and no lumps, can be consumed from a cup or spoon but not a fork.
- **Level 4 (Extremely thick)**: Liquids thickened to maintain their shape and need to be eaten with a spoon, not sticky, does not require chewing.

LEVELS OF SOLID TEXTURES

- **Level 3 (Liquidized)**: Same as Level 3 moderately thick above.
- **Level 4 (Pureed)**: Same as Level 4 extremely thick, above.
- **Level 5 (Minced and moist)**: Soft, visible lumps, can be consumed with a fork or spoon if lumps are easy to mash with tongue.
- **Level 6 (Soft and bite-sized)**: Soft-textured, moist, semi-solid foods that are easily chewed and swallowed.
- **Level 7**
  - **(Easy to chew)** Near-normal textured foods that are moist, can include mixed consistency. Hard, sticky foods are eliminated.
  - **(Regular)** Normal everyday foods, vary in texture, developmentally age appropriate.

NURSING ASSESSMENT/DATA COLLECTION AND INTERVENTIONS

- Ongoing assessment parameters include daily weights, prescribed laboratory tests, and an evaluation of a client's nutritional and energy needs and response to diet therapy.
- Observe and document nutritional intake. Perform a calorie count if needed to determine caloric intake and to evaluate adequacy.
- Provide education and support for diet therapy.
- A prescription for a diet as tolerated permits a client's preferences while taking into consideration the client's ability to eat. Assess the client for hunger, appetite, and nausea when planning the most appropriate diet, and consult with a dietitian.
- Dietary intake is progressively increased (from nothing by mouth to clear liquids to regular diet) following a major surgery. Nurses should assess for the return of bowel function (as evidenced by auscultation of bowel sounds and the passage of flatus) before advancing a client's diet. ⓠEBP

Active Learning Scenario

A nurse is planning care for a newly admitted client who has a prescription for a regular diet. Use the ATI Active Learning Template: Basic Concept to complete this item to include the following sections:

UNDERLYING PRINCIPLES: Identify the indication for a regular diet.

NURSING INTERVENTIONS

- Identify at least two assessments that are appropriate to determine the need for dietary modifications to the regular diet.
- Identify at least two nursing actions that are appropriate to monitor the client's response to diet therapy.

Application Exercises

1. A nurse is caring for a client following an appendectomy who has a postoperative prescription that reads "discontinue NPO status; advance diet to clear liquids as tolerated." Which of the following choices should the nurse offer the client? (Select all that apply.)

   A. Applesauce

   B. Chicken broth

   C. Sherbet

   D. Wheat toast

   E. Cranberry juice

   F. Granola

2. A nurse is performing dietary needs assessments for a group of clients. For which of the following clients should the nurse plan to provide a blenderized liquid diet? (Select all that apply.)

   A. A client who has a wired jaw due to a motor vehicle crash

   B. A client who is 24 hr postoperative following temporomandibular joint repair

   C. A client who has difficulty chewing due to oral surgery

   D. A client who has hypercholesterolemia due to coronary artery disease

   E. A client who is scheduled for a colonoscopy the next morning

3. A nurse is assisting a client who has a prescription for a mechanical soft diet with food selections. Which of the following are appropriate selections by the client? (Select all that apply.)

   A. Dried prunes

   B. Ground turkey

   C. Mashed carrots

   D. Fresh strawberries

   E. Cottage cheese

4. A nurse is caring for a client who is to receive a Level 2 dysphagia diet due to a recent stroke. Which of the following dietary selections is most appropriate?

   A. Turkey sandwich

   B. Scrambled eggs

   C. Peanut butter crackers

   D. Granola

Application Exercises Key

1. B, E. **CORRECT:** When taking actions, the nurse should offer the postoperative client who has a prescription for a clear liquid diet chicken broth or cranberry juice which can both be considered clear liquids.

   Ⓝ *NCLEX® Connection: Basic Care and Comfort, Nutrition and Oral Hydration*

2. A, B, C. **CORRECT:** When generating solutions following a dietary needs assessment, the nurse should plan to provide a blenderized liquid diet for a client who has a wired jaw, for a client following oral surgery and for a client who has difficulty chewing.

   Ⓝ *NCLEX® Connection: Reduction of Risk Potential, Potential for Alterations in Body Systems*

3. B, C, E. **CORRECT:** When taking actions and assisting a client select correct food choices for a mechanical soft diet, the nurse should identify that ground meats, mashed carrots, and cottage cheese require minimal chewing before swallowing and are therefore correct for a mechanical soft diet..

   Ⓝ *NCLEX® Connection: Basic Care and Comfort, Nutrition and Oral Hydration*

4. B. **CORRECT:** When taking actions caring for a client who requires a level 5 diet dysphagia diet, the nurse should offer the client foods that are moist, soft, and tender, such as scrambled eggs.

   Ⓝ *NCLEX® Connection: Reduction of Risk Potential, Potential for Complications of Diagnostic Tests/Treatments/Procedures*

Active Learning Scenario Key

Using the ATI Active Learning Template: Basic Concept

UNDERLYING PRINCIPLES: A regular diet is indicated for clients who do not need dietary restrictions.

NURSING INTERVENTIONS

Assessments to determine the need for dietary modification
- Individual preferences
- Food habits
- Ethnic values or practices

Assessments to monitor the client's response to diet therapy
- Obtain daily weight
- Monitor laboratory values
- Monitor energy level
- Observe and document nutritional intake
- Evaluate understanding of diet therapy

Ⓝ *NCLEX® Connection: Physiological Adaptation, Illness Management*

CHAPTER 9 *Enteral Nutrition*

Enteral nutrition (EN) is used when a client cannot consume adequate nutrients and calories orally but has a gastrointestinal (GI) system that functions at least partially. EN is contraindicated when the GI tract is nonfunctional (paralytic ileus or intestinal obstruction).

EN is administered when a client has a condition (burns, trauma, prolonged intubation, eating disorders, radiation therapy, chemotherapy, liver or renal dysfunction, infection, inflammatory bowel disease) that hinders nutritional status. EN is also administered when a client has neuromuscular impairment and cannot chew or swallow food.

EN feeding or gavage feeding for an infant is used when an infant is too weak for sucking, unable to coordinate swallowing, and lacks a gag reflex. Gavage feeding is implemented to conserve energy when an infant is attempting to breast feed or bottle feed, but becomes fatigued, weak, or cyanotic.

EN consists of a commercial formula administered by a tube into the stomach or small intestine. Enteral feedings most closely utilize the body's own digestive and metabolic routes. EN can augment an oral diet or be the sole source of nutrition.

ENTERAL FEEDING ROUTES

A client's medical status and the anticipated length of time that a tube feeding will be required determine the type of tube used.

Nasoenteric tubes

Nasoenteric tubes are short-term (less than 3 to 4 weeks).
- **Nasogastric** (NG) tubes are passed through the nose to the stomach.
- **Nasoduodenal** tubes pass from the nose through the stomach and end in the duodenum.
- **Nasojejunal** tubes pass from the nose through the stomach and end in the jejunum.
- Nasoduodenal and nasojejunal tubes are used in clients who are at risk for aspiration or who have delayed gastric emptying (gastroparesis).
- For an infant, a feeding tube is inserted from the nares or mouth into the stomach. This flexible tube can remain taped in place for up to 30 days.

Ostomies

Ostomies are placed for clients requiring long-term enteral feeding, who are at high risk for aspiration or when a nasal obstruction makes insertion through the nose impossible. An ostomy is a surgically created opening (stoma); ostomies can be used to deliver feedings directly into the stomach or intestines.

Gastrostomy tubes are endoscopically or surgically inserted into the stomach.
- A percutaneous endoscopic gastrostomy (PEG) tube is placed with the aid of an endoscope.
- An alternative to the PEG tube is a skin-level gastrostomy tube, which is known as a low-profile gastrostomy device. It is more comfortable, longer lasting, and fully immersible in water. Checking for residual is more difficult with this device because of the close proximity of the button on the skin.
- Gastrostomy tube feedings are generally well-tolerated because the stomach chamber holds and releases feedings in a physiologic manner that promotes effective digestion. As a result, dumping syndrome is usually avoided.

Jejunostomy tubes are surgically inserted into the jejunal portion of the small intestine (jejunum).

ENTERAL FEEDING FORMULAS

- Commercial products are preferred over home-blended ingredients because the nutrient composition, consistency and safety can be better insured.
- Standard and elemental formulas are the two primary types of enteral feeding formulas available. They are categorized by the complexity of the proteins included.
- Other formula types include disease-specific (COPD, kidney disease, immunocompromise) and modular formulas that typically contain a single nutrient (protein, carbohydrates, fat).

Standard formulas

- Also called polymeric or intact, these formulas are composed of whole proteins (milk, meat, eggs) or protein isolates.
- They require a functioning gastrointestinal tract.
- Most provide 1 to 2 cal/mL.

Hydrolyzed formulas

- These formulas are made up of nutrients that are partially or fully hydrolyzed or broken down.
- These formulas are used for clients who have a partially functioning gastrointestinal tract, or those who have an impaired ability to digest and absorb foods (inflammatory bowel disease, liver failure, cystic fibrosis, pancreatic disorders, and short-gut syndrome).
- Most provide 1.0 to 1.5 cal/mL. High-calorie formulas provide 1.5 to 2.0 cal/mL. Partially hydrolyzed formulas provide other nutrients in simpler forms that require little or no digestion.

PACKAGING

Tube feedings can be packaged in cans or prefilled bags.

- Prefilled bags and administration tubing should be discarded every 24 hr or according to facility policy, even if they are not empty.
- Cans can be used to add formula to a generic bag to infuse via a pump, or for feedings directly from a syringe.

DETERMINING APPROPRIATE FORMULA

Caloric density determines the volume of the formula necessary to meet the caloric needs of a client (1.0 to 1.2 cal/mL).

Water content in formulas with 1.0 cal/mL should be 850 mL water per 1 L formula. Higher-calorie formulas have lower water content. The client might need additional free water to meet hydration needs.

Osmolality of the formula is determined by the number of dissolved particles of sugars, amino acids, and electrolytes.

- Osmolality is increased if the formula contains more digested protein.
- Hydrolyzed or partially hydrolyzed (predigested) formulas are higher in osmolality than standard formulas. They are also lactose-free.

Fiber and residue content

- Standard formulas are low in residue which makes them less likely to produce abdominal distention or gas. These products are optimal for clients who have been on bowel rest, are postoperative following bowel surgery, or have GI related disease processes. Hydrolyzed formulas are considered residue-free.
- Standard formulas that are enriched with fiber are recommended for clients who have constipation or diarrhea to normalize bowel movements.

The presence of other nutrients includes fats and carbohydrates, which can be modified according to a client's disease processes (respiratory disease, malabsorption, diabetes mellitus, kidney disease).

ENTERAL FEEDING DELIVERY METHODS

The delivery method is dependent on the type and location of the feeding tube, type of formula administered, and the client's medical status and GI function.

Continuous infusion method

Formula is administered at a continuous rate over a 24-hr period.

- Infusion pumps help ensure consistent flow rates.
- This method is recommended for critically ill clients because of its association with smaller residual volumes, and a lower risk of aspiration and diarrhea.
- Some facilities require measuring gastric residual volume (GRV) every 4 to 6 hr. Most facilities are moving away from this practice, as there is insufficient evidence to support it.
- Feeding tubes should be flushed with at least 30 mL of water every 4 hr to maintain tube patency and provide hydration.
- Check facility policy regarding withholding feedings for high gastric residual volume (GRV). Typically, the amount is more than 250 mL on two consecutive measurements for an adult or more than one-fourth the prescribed volume for children.

Cyclic feeding

- Formula is administered at a continuous rate for 8 to 20 hr, often during sleeping hours.
- Often used for transition from total EN to oral intake.

Intermittent tube feeding

Formula is administered every 4 to 6 hr in equal portions, typically over a 30- to 60-min time frame, usually by gravity drip or an electronic pump. Feeding times can range from 20 to 90 min.

- This is often used for noncritical clients, home tube feedings, and clients in rehabilitation.
- Feeding resembles normal pattern of nutrient intake.
- Facilities might require measurement prior to initiating the feeding and held if the amount is greater than the amount stated in facility policy or prescription.

Bolus feeding

A variation of intermittent feeding using a large syringe attached to the feeding tube. The rate of administration and volume varies depending upon the client's needs and tolerance. Volumes ranging from 250 to 400 mL can be administered over a period of at least 15 min four to six times daily. Facility policies may provide further guidance regarding administration rates.

- The rate of administration for a premature or small infant should be no greater than 5 mL every 10 min, and 10 mL/min in older infants and children.
- Bolus feedings are delivered directly into the stomach; they are contraindicated for tubes placed into the jejunum or duodenum. They can be poorly tolerated and can cause dumping syndrome.

NURSING ACTIONS

PREPARATION OF THE CLIENT

- Prior to instilling enteral feeding, tube placement should be verified by radiography. The tube should then be marked with indelible ink or adhesive tape where it exits the nose and documented.
- Measure the tube each shift and prior to each feeding to ensure the tube has not migrated. Aspirating gastric contents and measuring pH levels are not considered reliable methods of verifying initial placement. Q EBP
- Verify the presence of bowel sounds.
- To maintain feeding tube patency, it is flushed routinely with warm water.
- Check gastric residuals if required by the facility, typically every 4 to 6 hr. In some cases, policy or prescription will indicate whether to return the contents to the client's stomach or to hold or reduce feedings.
  - The volume that indicates a need for intervention for adults ranges from 100 to 500 mL in a single measurement, or at least 250 mL on two consecutive checks.
  - Returning residual contents to the stomach prevents electrolyte and fluid imbalance. However, returning large volumes could increase the risk for complications.
- The head of the bed should be elevated at least 30° during feedings and for at least 30 to 60 min afterward to lessen the risk of aspiration. Q s
- Burp the infant following the feeding if the infant's condition allows.
- Begin with a small volume of full-strength formula. Increase volume in intervals as tolerated until the desired volume is achieved.
- Administer the feeding solution at room temperature to decrease gastrointestinal discomfort.
- Do not heat formulas in a microwave as this can result in uneven temperatures within the solution.

BASELINE PARAMETERS
- Obtain height, weight, and body mass index.
- Monitor blood urea nitrogen (BUN), albumin, hemoglobin, hematocrit, glucose, and electrolyte levels.
- A registered dietitian will work with the provider to evaluate nutritional and energy needs.
- Verify gastrointestinal function. Dysfunction of the GI tract can indicate a need for alternate forms of nutrition.

ONGOING CARE

- Monitor daily weights and I&O.
- Obtain gastric residuals every 4 to 6 hr.
- Monitor electrolytes, BUN, creatinine, minerals, and CBC.
- Monitor the tube site for manifestations of infection or intolerance (pain, redness, swelling, drainage).
- Monitor the character and frequency of bowel movements.

- When appropriate, administer medications through a feeding tube.
  - Feeding should be stopped prior to administering medications.
  - The tubing should be flushed with water (15 to 30 mL) before and after the medication is administered, and between each medication if more than one is administered.
  - Medications should only be dissolved in water.
  - Liquid medications should be used when possible.
    - For an infant or child, the volume of water to flush is 1.5 times the amount predetermined to flush an unused feeding tube of the same size.
    - More water can be required to flush the tubing following some medications (suspensions).

INTERVENTIONS

- Weaning occurs as oral consumption increases. Enteral feedings can be discontinued when the client consumes two-thirds of protein and calorie needs orally for 3 to 5 days.
- A client who is NPO will require meticulous oral care.
- A client can require nutritional support service at home for long-term EN. A interprofessional team comprised of a nurse, dietitian, pharmacist, and the provider monitors the client's weight, electrolyte balance, and overall physical condition. Q TC
- Transitioning from EN to an oral diet requires the client to receive adequate nutrition as food items are reintroduced.
  - Begin the transition process by stopping the EN for 1 hr before a meal.
  - Slowly increase the frequency of the meals until the client is eating up to six small meals daily.
  - When oral intake equals 500 to 750 cal/day, the continuous tube feeding is administered only during the night.

COMPLICATIONS

Gastrointestinal complications

- Constipation, diarrhea, cramping, pain, abdominal distention, dumping syndrome, nausea, and vomiting.
- Dumping syndrome occurs due to rapid emptying of the formula into the small intestine, resulting in a fluid shift. Manifestations include dizziness, rapid pulse, diaphoresis, pallor, and lightheadedness.

NURSING ACTIONS
- Consider a change in formula.
- Decrease the flow rate or total volume of the infusion.
- Increase the volume of free water if constipated.
- Administer the EN at room temperature.
- Take measures to prevent bacterial contamination.

Mechanical complications

Tube misplacement or dislodgement; aspiration; irritation and leakage at the insertion site; irritation of the nose, esophagus, and mucosa; and clogging of the feeding tube.

NURSING ACTIONS
- Confirm tube placement prior to feedings.
- Elevate the head of the bed at least 30° during feedings and maintain the client in this position for approximately 60 min following completion of the feeding.
- Administer bolus feedings over a period of at least 15 min and according to client tolerance.
- Flush the tubing with at least 30 mL of water every 4 hr for continuous infusion, after measuring gastric residual, before and after bolus feedings, and between each medication administration.
- Unclog tubing using gentle pressure with 30 to 50 mL warm water in a 60 mL piston syringe. Carbonated beverages are not approved for fixing a clogged tube. Commercially made products are available and have been shown to effectively dissolve clotted formula.
- Do not mix medications with the formula.

Metabolic complications

Include dehydration, hyperglycemia, electrolyte imbalances, fluid overload, refeeding syndrome, rapid weight gain

NURSING ACTIONS
- Provide adequate amounts of free water.
- Consider changing formula to one that is isotonic.
- Restrict fluids if fluid overload occurs.
- Monitor electrolytes, blood glucose, and weights.
- Monitor respiratory, cardiovascular, and neurologic status.
- Administer insulin per prescribed protocol for hyperglycemia.

Refeeding syndrome

A potentially fatal complication that occurs when a client who is in a starvation state is started on enteral nutrition. The risk is greater with parenteral nutrition than enteral.

Foodborne illness

Can result due to bacterial contamination of formula

NURSING ACTIONS: Prevent bacterial contamination.
- Wash hands before handling formula or enteral products.
- Clean equipment and tops of formula cans.
- Use closed feeding systems.
- Cover and label open cans with unused portions with the client's name, room number, date, and time of opening.
- Replace the feeding bag, administration tubing, and any equipment used to mix the formula every 24 hr.
- Fill generic bags with only 4 hr worth of formula.

Application Exercises

1. A nurse is discussing the use of a low-profile, or skin-level, gastrostomy device with the guardian of a child who is receiving an enteral feeding. Which of the following statements should the nurse make?
    A. "The device is usually comfortable for children."
    B. "Checking residual is much easier with this device."
    C. "This access requires less maintenance than a traditional nasal tube."
    D. "Mobility of the child is limited with this device."

2. A nurse is teaching a client who is starting continuous feedings about the various types of enteral nutrition (EN) formulas. Which of the following should the nurse include in the teaching?
    A. Formula rich in fiber is recommended when starting EN.
    B. Standard formula contains whole protein.
    C. Hydrolyzed formula is recommended for a full-functioning GI tract.
    D. The high-calorie formula has increased water content.

3. A nurse is instructing a client about administering cyclic enteral feedings at home. Which of the following information should the nurse include? (Select all that apply.)
    A. "Give a feeding every 6 hours."
    B. "Set the feeding up before you go to bed."
    C. "Weigh yourself daily."
    D. "Flush the tube with a carbonated beverage to dislodge clogs."
    E. "Ensure your head is elevated to 15 degrees during administration."

4. A nurse is preparing to administer intermittent enteral feedings to a client. Which of the following actions should the nurse plan to take? (Select all that apply.)
    A. Fill the feeding bag with 24 hr worth of formula.
    B. Discard feeding equipment after 24 hr.
    C. Ensure that the formula is at room temperature.
    D. Flush the feeding tube every 4 hr.
    E. Elevate the head of the client's bed for 15 min after administration.

5. A nurse is administering bolus enteral feedings to a client who has malnutrition. Which of the following are appropriate nursing interventions? (Select all that apply.)
    A. Verify the presence of bowel sounds.
    B. Flush the feeding tube with warm water.
    C. Elevate the head of the bed 20°.
    D. Administer the feeding at room temperature.
    E. Instill the formula over 60 min.

Application Exercises Key

1. A. **CORRECT:** When taking actions, the nurse should inform the guardian that a gastrostomy device is longer-lasting and is more comfortable for children because of the proximity of the button on the skin.

   Ⓝ *NCLEX® Connection: Basic Care and Comfort, Nutrition and Oral Hydration*

2. B. **CORRECT:** When taking actions, the nurse should teach the client that a standard formula contains whole protein (milk, meat, eggs) and requires a full-functioning GI tract.

   Ⓝ *NCLEX® Connection: Basic Care and Comfort, Nutrition and Oral Hydration*

3. B, C. **CORRECT:** Many clients administer cyclic feedings during sleeping hours, so they are free during the daytime to do other things.

   Ⓝ *NCLEX® Connection: Basic Care and Comfort, Nutrition and Oral Hydration*

4. B, C, D. **CORRECT:** When generating solutions regarding the administration of enteral feedings to a client, the nurse should plan to discard the feeding equipment, such as the bag holding the formula and the tubing, every 24 hr to prevent bacterial contamination. The nurse should also plan to have the formula at room temperature prior to administration and be prepared to flush the feeding tube immediately following the feeding to maintain patency..

   Ⓝ *NCLEX® Connection: Basic Care and Comfort, Nutrition and Oral Hydration*

5. A, B, D. **CORRECT:** When taking actions and administering a bolus enteral feeding to a client, the nurse should verify the presence of bowel sounds prior to the feeding to ensure the bowel is functioning as well as flushing the feeding tube to ensure patency. The nurse should administer the bolus feeding at room temperature to prevent abdominal cramping

   Ⓝ *NCLEX® Connection: Basic Care and Comfort, Nutrition and Oral Hydration*

Active Learning Scenario

A nurse is providing information to a client on complications that can occur when administering an enteral nutrition. What information should the nurse include in the teaching? Use the ATI Active Learning Template: Basic Concept to complete this item to include the following.

RELATED CONTENT: Identify three complications. List two nursing interventions for each complication.

Active Learning Scenario Key

Using the ATI Active Learning Template: Basic Concept
RELATED CONTENT

Gastrointestinal disturbance
• Increase the amount of free fluid if constipated.
• Consider a change to formula with enriched fiber if constipated.
• Decrease the flow rate if cramping occurs.
• Give the formula at room temperature.

Feeding tube obstruction
• Flush the tubing with at least 30 mL of water every 4 hr.
• Flush before and after feedings and medication.
• Use a piston syringe with 50 mL of warm water to unclog the tubing.
• Carbonated beverages are not approved to clear clogged enteral tubes.

Foodborne illness
• Wash hands before handling the formula or equipment.
• Clean tops of formula containers.
• Cover and refrigerate formula up to 24 hr.
• Replace the feeding bag and administration tubing every 24 hr.

Ⓝ *NCLEX® Connection: Reduction of Risk Potential, Potential for Complications of Diagnostic Tests/Treatments/Procedures*

UNIT 2   CLINICAL NUTRITION

CHAPTER 10 *Total Parenteral Nutrition*

Parenteral nutrition (PN) is used when a client's gastrointestinal tract is not functioning, or when a client cannot physically or psychologically consume sufficient nutrients orally or enterally. Based upon the client's nutritional needs and anticipated duration of therapy, PN can be given as either total parenteral nutrition (TPN) or peripheral parenteral nutrition (PPN).

TPN provides a nutritionally complete solution. It can be used when caloric needs are very high, when long-term therapy is indicated, or when the solution to be administered is hypertonic (composed of greater than 10% dextrose). It can only be administered in a central vein.

PPN is administered for 7 to 10 days into a peripheral vein. It is nutritionally incomplete because it has a low dextrose content. It is indicated for clients who require short-term nutritional support with fewer calories per day. The solution must be isotonic and contain no more than 10% dextrose and 5% amino acids.

COMPONENTS OF PARENTERAL NUTRITION SOLUTIONS

PN includes amino acids, dextrose, electrolytes, vitamins, and trace elements in sterile water. Fats (lipids) are added to the parenteral solution or given as an intermittent infusion.

Carbohydrate or dextrose solutions are available in concentrations of 2.5% to 10% for PPN and up to 70% for TPN.
- A higher concentration of dextrose is often prescribed for a client on fluid restrictions.
- A lower-dextrose concentration can be used to help control hyperglycemia.

Electrolytes, vitamins, and trace elements are essential for normal body functions. The amounts added are dependent upon the client's blood chemistry values and physical findings, which are used to determine the quantity of electrolytes. Additional vitamin K can be added to the PN solution.

Lipids (fats) are available in concentrations of 10%, 20%, and 30%. Lipids are formulated from a combination of soybean oil and/or safflower oil, and egg phospholipids, which gives lipids a milky or opaque appearance.
- IV lipids are contraindicated for clients who have severe hyperlipidemia, severe hepatic disease, or an allergy to soybean oil, eggs, or safflower oil.
- Lipid emulsion provides the needed calories when dextrose concentration must be reduced due to fluid restrictions or persistent hyperglycemia. They also correct or prevent essential fatty acid deficiency.
- Lipid emulsion provides the calories without increasing the osmolality of the PN solution.
- Total nutrient admixtures are available that combine lipids into the PN solution containing dextrose and amino acids, rather than administering the solutions separately. Not all facilities use this three-in-one solution.
  - Three-in-one infusions reduce body carbon dioxide production and buildup of fat in the liver.

Protein is provided as a mixture of essential and nonessential amino acids and is available in concentrations of 3% to 20%. The client's estimated requirements and liver and kidney function determine the amount of protein provided.

Other substances can be added to the PN solution by pharmacy services.
- Insulin can be added to reduce the potential for hyperglycemia.
- Heparin can be added to prevent fibrin buildup on the catheter tip.
- Glutamine, antioxidants, prebiotics, or probiotics might be prescribed based on individual client needs.

! Administering any IV medication through a PN IV line or port is contraindicated.

INDICATIONS

DIAGNOSES

- TPN is commonly used in clients who need intense nutritional support for an extended period, including clients undergoing treatment for cancer, bowel disorders, those who are critically ill, and those suffering from trauma or extensive burns, as these conditions are associated with high caloric requirements.
- PPN can be used when the client is unable to consume enough calories to meet metabolic needs or when nutritional support is needed for a short time.
- Clients can receive PN at home as nutrition replacement or to supplement nutrition. Typically, the client will have a tunneled catheter, and feedings can occur while the client sleeps.

DESIRED THERAPEUTIC OUTCOMES

- Improved nutritional status
- Weight maintenance or gain
- Positive nitrogen balance

EVIDENCE SUPPORTING EFFECTIVENESS

- Daily weight: Maintenance of baseline or gain of up to 1 kg/day
- Increases in prealbumin level (expected reference range of 15 to 36 mg/dL)
- Blood urea nitrogen level within the expected reference range (10 to 20 mg/dL)

CONSIDERATIONS

PREPARATION OF THE CLIENT

- Prior to initiating PN, review the client's weight, BMI, nutritional status, diagnosis, and current laboratory data. This can include CBC, blood chemistry profile, PT/aPTT, iron, total iron-binding capacity, lipid profile, liver function tests, electrolyte panel, BUN, prealbumin and albumin level, creatinine, blood glucose, and platelet count.
- Assess the client's educational needs.
- Use an electronic infusion device to prevent the accidental overload of a solution.
- A micron filter on the IV tubing is required when administering PN solution. This filter is not added to the IV tubing when administering a lipid emulsion.
- Evaluate for allergies to soybeans, safflower, or eggs if lipids are prescribed.

ONGOING CARE

Nursing care is focused on preventing complications through consistent monitoring. Specific monitoring guidelines vary among health care facilities.

- Parameters can include I&O, daily weights, vital signs, pertinent laboratory values (e.g., electrolytes), and evaluation of the client's underlying condition. This data is used to determine the client's response to therapy, whether the formulation of the solution is correct, and to prevent nutrient deficiencies or toxicities.
- Monitor blood and urine glucose as prescribed and per facility guidelines. Sliding scale insulin can treat or prevent hyperglycemia, or regular insulin can be added to the PN solution.
- Monitor flow rate carefully.
  - Administering the solution too slowly will fail to meet the client's nutritional needs.
  - Administering the infusion too rapidly can cause hyperosmolar diuresis, which can lead to dehydration, hypovolemic shock, seizures, coma, and death.
  - To avoid hypoglycemia, an IV of dextrose 10% to 20% in water is administered if the PN solution is unavailable.
  - Do not attempt to increase the rate of the PN solution to "catch up." Hyperglycemia, hyperosmolar diuresis, and fluid overload can occur if the PN solution is increased when available.

- Monitor for "cracking" of TPN solution. This occurs if the calcium or phosphorous content is high or if poor-salt albumin is added. A "cracked" TPN solution has an oily appearance or a layer of fat on top of the solution and should not be used. Qs
- Verify the prescription of the PN solution with a second nurse prior to administration.
- If the PN solution is prepared and stored in the refrigerator, allow it to come to room temperature for 1 hr prior to administering it.
- Maintain strict aseptic techniques to reduce the risk of infection. The high dextrose content of PN contributes to bacterial growth. QSDoH
- Use sterile technique when changing central line dressing and tubing. Change the bag and IV tubing for the dextrose solution every 24 hr unless facility policy differs. With intermittent IV lipid infusions, ensure the solution does not hang more than 12 hr to prevent microbial growth.
- Ensure lipid infusion is stopped 12 hr prior to obtaining a blood specimen for triglycerides to ensure accurate results.

NURSING ACTIONS

- Ask the provider about giving some enteral substance during long-term PN administration, such as diluted juice, to prevent atrophy of the gastrointestinal tract. QEBP
- PN should be discontinued as soon as possible to avoid potential complications, but not until the client's enteral or oral intake can provide 50% to 75% of estimated caloric requirements.

  !Discontinuation should be done gradually to avoid rebound hypoglycemia.

- During transition, the client will need enteral or oral nutrition. Oral nutrition usually begins with clear liquids that are low in fat or substances that might irritate the client's gastrointestinal tract. The client might not have an appetite for 1 to 2 weeks, so PN infusion will need to continue until the client can take in adequate calories through other means.
- Educate the client and family regarding home PN, including aseptic preparation and administration techniques, blood glucose monitoring, and criteria to evaluate for complications.

COMPLICATIONS

Infection and sepsis are evidenced by a fever or elevated WBC count. Infection can result from contamination of the catheter during insertion, contaminated solution, or a long-term indwelling catheter.

Metabolic complications include hyperglycemia, hypoglycemia, hyperkalemia, hypophosphatemia, hypocalcemia, dehydration (related to hyperosmolar diuresis resulting from hyperglycemia), and fluid overload (as evidenced by weight gain greater than 1 kg/day and edema).

Mechanical complications include catheter misplacement resulting in pneumothorax or hemothorax (evidenced by shortness of breath, diminished or absent breath sounds), arterial puncture, catheter embolus, air embolus, thrombosis, obstruction, and bolus infusion due to incorrectly set or malfunctioning electronic pumps.

Refeeding syndrome occurs when the body rapidly changes from catabolic (seen in starvation states) to anabolic metabolism when nutrition is started. It is characterized by fluid and electrolyte imbalances (potassium, magnesium, phosphate). Manifestations include shallow respirations, confusion, seizures, weakness, cardiac rhythm changes, fluid retention, and acidosis.

NURSING ACTIONS

- Monitor for manifestations of fever, chills, increased WBCs, and redness around the catheter insertion site.
- Use strict aseptic technique when setting up the IV tubing, changing the site dressing, and accessing or deaccessing the IV access. Change the PN bag and tubing set every 24 hr or per facility protocol.
- Monitor blood glucose per prescription or facility policy.
- Administer sliding scale insulin or plan for insulin to be added to the TPN solution to treat hyperglycemia.
- Plan to administer additional dextrose to treat hypoglycemia.
- Monitor daily weights, I&O, and oral intake of nutrients.
- Notify the provider of weight gain greater than 1 kg/day.
- Anticipate a decrease in the concentration of the solution, rate of administration, or volume of lipid emulsion to treat weight gain.

Active Learning Scenario

A nurse is teaching a client about complications that can occur when receiving total parenteral nutrition (TPN). What should the nurse include in the teaching? Use the ATI Active Learning Template: Basic Concept to complete this item to include the following.

RELATED CONTENT: Identify three complications of TPN. Describe two nursing actions related to each complication.

Application Exercises

1. A charge nurse is providing information about fat emulsion added to total parenteral nutrition (TPN) to a group of nurses. Which of the following information should the charge nurse include? (Select all that apply.)
   A. "Concentration of lipid emulsion can be up to 30%."
   B. "Adding lipid emulsion gives the solution a milky appearance."
   C. "Check for allergies to soybean oil."
   D. "Lipid emulsion prevents essential fatty acid deficiency."
   E. "Lipids provide calories by increasing the osmolality of the PN solution."

2. A charge nurse is teaching a group of nurses about medication compatibility with TPN. Which of the following statements should the charge nurse make?
   A. "Use the Y-port on the TPN IV tubing to administer antibiotics."
   B. "Regular insulin can be added to the TPN solution."
   C. "Administer heparin through a port on the TPN tubing."
   D. "Administer vitamin K IV bolus via a Y-port on the TPN tubing."

3. A nurse is preparing to administer lipid emulsion and notes a layer of fat floating in the IV solution bag. Which of the following actions should the nurse take?
   A. Shake the bag to mix the fat.
   B. Turn the bag upside down one time.
   C. Return the bag to the pharmacy.
   D. Administer the bag of solution as it is.

4. A nurse is caring for a client who is receiving TPN through a central venous access device, but the next bag of solution is not available for administration at this time. Which of the following is actions should the nurse take?
   A. Administer 20% dextrose in water IV until the next bag is available.
   B. Slow the infusion rate of the current bag until the solution is available.
   C. Monitor for hyperglycemia.
   D. Monitor for hyperosmolar diuresis.

5. A nurse is planning care for a client who has a new prescription for peripheral parenteral nutrition (PPN). Which of the following actions should the nurse include in the plan of care? (Select all that apply.)
   A. Examine trends in weight loss.
   B. Review prealbumin finding.
   C. Administer an IV solution of 20% dextrose.
   D. Use IV tubing with a micron filter.
   E. Use an IV infusion pump.

Active Learning Scenario Key

Using the ATI Active Learning Template: Basic Concept

RELATED CONTENT

Infection and sepsis

- Monitor for manifestations of fever, chills, increased WBCs, and redness around catheter insertion site.
- Use aseptic technique when setting up the IV tubing and accessing or deaccessing the port.
- Use sterile technique when changing central line dressing and tubing.
- Change the PN bag and tubing set every 24 hr or per facility protocol.

Hyperglycemia

- Administer sliding scale insulin or plan for insulin to be added to the TPN solution.
- Monitor blood glucose.

Hypoglycemia

- Inform the provider and plan to give additional dextrose.
- Monitor frequent blood glucose.

Weight gain greater than 1 kg/day

- Inform the provider and anticipate a decrease in the concentration, rate of administration or volume of lipid emulsion.
- Monitor the client's intake of oral nutrients.

Ⓝ *NCLEX® Connection: Pharmacological and Parenteral Therapies, Nutrition and Oral Hydration*

Application Exercises Key

1. A, B, C, D. **CORRECT:** When taking actions and providing information to other nurses about lipid emulsions, the nurse should include that lipid emulsion is available in 10%, 20%, and 30% concentrations and can be formulated from safflower and/or soybean oils and egg phospholipids, making the solution appear milky. When administering a lipid emulsion formulated from safflower and/or soybean oil and egg phospholipids, the nurse should check for allergies to these ingredients. Lipid emulsion is used for additional calories as concentrated energy and to prevent essential fatty acid deficiency.

   Ⓝ *NCLEX® Connection: Pharmacological and Parenteral Therapies, Total Parenteral Nutrition*

2. B. **CORRECT:** When taking actions and teaching nurses about medication compatibility with TPN, the nurse should state that regular insulin can be added to the TPN solution to decrease hyperglycemia.

   Ⓝ *NCLEX® Connection: Pharmacological and Parenteral Therapies, Total Parenteral Nutrition*

3. C. **CORRECT:** When generating solutions preparing to administer a lipid emulsion to a client, the nurse should return the solution to the pharmacy if cracking of the solution has occurred, and it should not be administered.

   Ⓝ *NCLEX® Connection: Pharmacological and Parenteral Therapies, Nutrition and Oral Hydration*

4. A. **CORRECT:** When generating solutions for a client receiving TPN and whose next bag of solution is not available, the nurse should plan to administer 20% dextrose in water IV until the TPN solution is available to reduce the risk of developing hypoglycemia.

   Ⓝ *NCLEX® Connection: Pharmacological and Parenteral Therapies, Total Parenteral Nutrition*

5. A, B, D, E. **CORRECT:** The nurse should plan to generate solutions and plan care for a client who has a prescription for PPN which includes examining trends in weight loss to evaluate the outcome of PPN, reviewing the prealbumin level to determine nutritional deficiency over a short period of time, using tubing with a micron filter when infusing PN solution, and using an IV infusion pump to regulate the flow and provide accurate delivery of the PN solution.

   Ⓝ *NCLEX® Connection: Pharmacological and Parenteral Therapies, Total Parenteral Nutrition*

When reviewing the following chapters, keep in mind the relevant topics and tasks of the NCLEX outline, in particular:

Health Promotion and Maintenance

HEALTH PROMOTION/DISEASE PREVENTION
Identify risk factors for disease/illness.

Educate the client on actions to promote/maintain health and prevent disease.

HEALTH SCREENING: Perform targeted screening assessments.

HIGH-RISK BEHAVIORS: Assist the client to identify behaviors/risks that may impact health.

Basic Care and Comfort

ELIMINATION: Assess and manage client with an alteration in elimination.

NUTRITION AND ORAL HYDRATION
Provide nutritional supplements as needed.

Evaluate the impact of disease/illness on the nutritional status of a client.

Physiological Adaptation

ALTERATIONS IN BODY SYSTEMS: Implement interventions to address side/adverse effects of radiation therapy.

ILLNESS MANAGEMENT: Educate the client about managing illness.

FLUID AND ELECTROLYTE IMBALANCES: Manage the care of the client who has a fluid and electrolyte imbalance.

Reduction of Risk Potential

POTENTIAL FOR ALTERATIONS IN BODY SYSTEMS: Identify client potential for aspiration.

SYSTEM-SPECIFIC ASSESSMENTS: Assess the client for signs of hypoglycemia or hyperglycemia.

UNIT 3   ALTERATIONS IN NUTRITION

CHAPTER 11   *Barriers to Adequate Nutrition*

Many individuals have difficulty consuming a nutritional or prescribed diet due to factors that create a barrier. Medical, psychological, and social factors can all create nutritional barriers. Approximately 30% to 50% of clients in acute care facilities are malnourished upon admission or during part of their hospital stay.

It is important for nurses to recognize these factors, as nutritional education will be ineffective if a client lacks the necessary resources to follow through on recommendations.

NUTRITIONAL BARRIERS AND NURSING INTERVENTIONS

Poor dentition

Poor dentition (dental caries, poorly fitting dentures) is a potential problem for clients across the lifespan.
- Children who do not have access to dental care or tools (toothbrush, toothpaste) can have caries that impair the ability to chew.
- Adults who have lost teeth or have teeth that need removal or repair have an impaired ability to chew.
- After an adult has teeth removed, it can be difficult to adjust to dentures.

NURSING CARE
- School screenings can help identify children who need dental attention and can facilitate the referral process.
- Provide children with information about healthy snacks that are low in sugar.
- Advise children and adults to limit consumption of processed carbohydrates, which can stick to teeth and increase the risk for dental caries.
- Encourage children and adults to use a fluoridated tooth paste and have fluoride applied to their teeth. Q͏EBP
- Perform a basic dental screening for clients admitted to acute or long-term care facilities to identify issues that can affect the ability to properly eat.
- Consult a dietitian or nutritionist to assist with meal and diet planning, as well as for recommendations on nutritional supplements. Q͏TC

Low socioeconomic status and lack of access Q͏SDoH

The lack of money to purchase healthy foods or foods required for a specific diet can be a barrier to maintaining a proper diet.
- Nutritious foods (fresh fruit, vegetables) tend to be more expensive than canned and boxed foods.
- Canned, boxed, and processed foods (lunch meats and frozen meals) are usually high in calories and salt, and often contain a higher fat, sodium, and simple carbohydrate content. These are poor choices for clients on calorie- or sodium-restricted diets.
- The lack of money to purchase necessary food can lead to malnutrition or obesity if canned and boxed foods are selected.
- The lack of transportation to grocery stores is a barrier if the client does not have a car or is not licensed to drive.
- Food deserts occur in low-socioeconomic areas where a person lives more than 1 mile from a food source in the urban area, or more than 10 miles in a rural area.
- Groups with higher-than-average rates of food insecurity:
  ○ Households with incomes near or below the poverty line
  ○ Families in which the head of the household is a single parent
  ○ Families in which the head of the household is Black or Hispanic
  ○ Households in large metropolitan areas

NURSING CARE
- Refer the client to a dietitian who can discuss food options and substitutions that are appropriate.
- Instruct the client that frozen fruits and vegetables can be an affordable option and are maintained longer in the freezer.
- Educate clients on how to read food labels to be aware of nutritional, caloric, and sodium values of the food they are consuming.
- Contact social services regarding the client's access to food. Investigate the availability of a nutrition program that provides a meal for clients within a community. Q͏S

Cognitive disorders

Cognitive disorders (dementia, Alzheimer's disease [AD]) can have a significant impact on nutritional status.
- Clients who have dementia or AD can experience impairments in memory and judgment, making shopping, food selection, and food preparation difficult.
- As dementia and AD progress, clients might refuse to eat or choose a small selection of food that might not provide adequate nutrition.

NURSING CARE

- If the client lives independently, encourage shopping with a friend or family member and following a shopping list.
- Monitor for vitamin and mineral deficits and evaluate the need for nutritional supplements.
- Contact social services regarding the availability of food or meal delivery to the client's home.
- If the client lives in a care facility, provide a menu with minimal but nutritious options.
- Serve meals at the same time and in the same location surrounded by the same people. Keep environmental distractions to a minimum.
- Provide snacks in between meals if mealtime intake is inadequate.
- Cut food into small pieces if the client has difficulty chewing food. Remind the client to chew and then swallow. Lightly stroking the chin and throat can help promote swallowing. Qs

Altered sensory perception

Clients who have an alteration in vision, smell, or taste can find it difficult to feed themselves or can find food unpalatable.

- Clients who have decreased vision might need assistance shopping for food on a regular basis, and with food preparation.
- Clients in a health care or long-term care facility might need help with tray setup and location of food on the tray.
- Clients who have an altered sense of smell have an altered sense of taste.
- Clients who smoke might have a diminished sense of smell.
- Clients receiving chemotherapy and other types of medications can experience taste alterations such as a metallic taste in their mouth, masking the real taste of food.
- Clients receiving radiation to the head and neck can experience altered or loss of taste (mouth blindness).

11.1 Case Study

Scenario introduction

A nurse on the medical-surgical unit is caring for a client who has had a diagnosis of hypertension for two years. The client has been seen in the emergency department twice during the last 3 months for hypertension and headaches. The client was admitted with a blood pressure of 180/110 and a headache. Their BMI is 34. On admission, the client reported non-adherence with their plan for diet changes and antihypertensive medications.

Scene 1

The nurse and client are seated in the client's hospital room.

Nurse: While you are in the hospital, I would like to see how we can help you maintain better control of your blood pressure. Tell me how you take your blood pressure medications.

Client: I was taking them every day; however I was unable to get them refilled because my money ran out. I lost my job about 6 months ago, so I don't have insurance anymore. I never finished high school, so I don't have many job options.

Scene 2

The nurse and client continue to talk. The nurse has some sample menus and charts with nutrient values of foods.

Nurse: Let's talk about what kinds of foods you usually eat.

Client: Whatever I can get. When money is short, I buy a lot of canned food, because it's cheap, and I can eat it right out of the can without having to use electricity to cook. Sometimes my electricity gets turned off, so I can't use the stove or refrigerator. When I can, I buy inexpensive cuts of meat.

Nurse: I can see how your financial situation has impacted your lifestyle. I would like to explore some options with you to assist with meeting your needs. Do you know how to select healthy food options by being attentive to the food labels?

Client: No, I just purchase foods. I can read but not very well.

Scene 3

Nurse: I would like to have the dietitian talk with you before you are discharged to help you find ways to have more nutritious foods in your diet.

Client: Okay, but I saw a dietitian when I first found out I have high blood pressure. They didn't really seem to understand the way I eat. I don't think a lot of doctors and nurses here understand that where I come from, we eat a lot of meat, we cook with salt and fat. They tell me to stop eating those things and lose some weight, but they don't understand that's what I love to eat, and when you cook with those, you can get a lot of flavors without a lot of ingredients.

Scenario conclusion

The dietitian collaborates with the client and reviews healthier ways to buy and prepare foods. The dietitian uses educational materials with pictures and graphs. The nurse is planning to consult with other members of the interprofessional team to assist the client with meeting their needs to improve health outcomes.

Case study exercises

1. The nurse recognizes that the client has reported multiple factors that impact their health. Which of the following social determinants of health (SDOH) were mentioned by the client? (Select all that apply.)

   A. Economic stability

   B. Education access and quality

   C. Health care access and quality

   D. Neighborhood and built environment

   E. Social and community context

2. When preparing this client for discharge, the nurse includes the dietitian in planning. What other types of referrals should the nurse make to other members of the health care team? What kinds of resources might they help the client find?

3. What are some suggestions the interprofessional health care team can make to this client to assist with regularly checking their blood pressure and weight?

NURSING CARE

- Encourage the client who has decreased vision to consider shopping with a friend or family member, or have groceries delivered to the house. Qᴘᴄᴄ
- Contact social services regarding availability of food or meal delivery to the client's home.
- Recommend to the client who has a food aversion to eat foods that are served cool, as they are typically less aromatic and are less likely to precipitate nausea.
- Suggest consuming foods that are spicy or tangy to compensate for the decreased sense of taste.
- Recommend sucking on hard candies, mints, or chewing gum to counteract an unusual taste in the mouth.
- Instruct the client to avoid ingestion of empty calories. If an increase in calories and fluid is desired, milkshakes, juice, and supplements are good options.

Impairment in swallowing

Clients who have neurologic disorders (Parkinson's disease, cerebral palsy, stroke) or had a surgical procedure done on their mouth, throat, epiglottis, or larynx can have difficulty managing food and swallowing without choking.

- Clients who have a neurologic disorder affecting the muscles in the mouth and throat are at risk for aspiration due to delayed swallowing and/or inadequate mastication.
- Clients who have a history of oral cancer might have had part of their lip, tongue, and/or soft palate removed. This significantly affects the ability to masticate and coordinate the development of a bolus of food prior to swallowing.
- The larynx and epiglottis prevent food from entering the trachea. Clients who have had partial removal of the larynx can easily aspirate food and fluids, unless special precautions are taken. A client who has had a total laryngectomy cannot aspirate food, because the airway and esophagus are separated.

NURSING CARE

- Continually monitor clients who are at risk for aspiration during meals, and have suction equipment immediately available. Qꜱ
- Consult a dietitian regarding an appropriate diet for the client. The National Dysphagia diet includes three levels of solid textures.
  - Level 1: Pureed
  - Level 2: Mechanically altered
  - Level 3: Advanced
- Thicken thin fluids with a commercial thickener to the prescribed consistency of thin, nectar-like, honey-like, or spoon-thick.
- Allow adequate time for assisting the client who has dysphagia to eat. Have the client rest before meals.
- Teach clients who aspirate easily due to surgical alteration of their throat or upper tracheal structures to tuck their chins when swallowing. Arching the tongue in the back of the throat can help close off the trachea.

Mechanical fixation of the jaw

Disorders of the jaw requiring surgery include facial trauma and reconstruction.

- After fractured bones are realigned, the client's upper and lower jaw might be wired together.
- The jaw can be immobilized for several weeks.
- The client is generally placed on a liquid diet during this period.

NURSING CARE

- Encourage the intake of fluids.
- Help the client determine where to insert a straw through the space between the jaws.
- Work with the dietitian to develop a liquid meal plan that includes the necessary nutrients. Qᴛᴄ

Lack of knowledge and misinformation about nutrition

Clients can be subject to overnutrition, undernutrition, and the ingestion of an inadequate intake of essential nutrients.

- Clients might not have basic knowledge about nutrition.
- Information about nutrition can be confusing or misleading.
- Clients can be drawn to fad diets (which are generally unhealthy) because quick results are promised.
- Clients can be misled by false advertising.

NURSING CARE

- Encourage clients to use dietary guidelines available from government and health associations (MyPlate, American Heart Association, Office of Disease Prevention and Health Promotion Dietary Guidelines). Qᴇʙᴘ
- Assist clients in locating community resources that provide education on nutrition.
- Assess dietary intake.
- Instruct clients on how to read nutrition fact labels.
- Encourage the client to keep a journal of dietary intake.
- Provide clients with information on foods that are healthy and portion sizes.
- Warn clients that advertisements can be fraudulent.

Medical conditions

- Clients who have medical conditions (cancer, COPD, burns, severe trauma, or HIV/AIDS) are at increased risk for malnutrition due to anorexia, nausea, or stomatitis related to treatments, increased metabolic demands, or the inability to consume a diet.
- Clients who are undergoing diagnostic testing that require NPO status are potentially at risk.
- Clients who have comorbidities resulting in polypharmacy are at risk for malnutrition and medication nutrient interactions.

NURSING CARE

- Monitor diet prescriptions and laboratory results, particularly for clients who are NPO or are receiving clear or full liquid diets for more than 24 hr. Refer the client to a dietitian for a complete evaluation of nutritional status. Qℝᴄ
- Monitor clients who have comorbidities for interactions between medications and nutrition. Refer the client to a pharmacist for a thorough evaluation of medication interactions and the impact upon nutritional intake.
- Offer several small meals or snacks through the day instead of three large meals if the client cannot tolerate large amounts at once.
- Provide oral care prior to and following meals.
- Discourage the use of alcohol-based mouthwashes for clients who have stomatitis.
- Provide liquid supplements between meals to increase nutrient intake.

Case Study Exercises Key

1. A, B, C, E. **CORRECT:** When analyzing cues, the nurse should determine that the SDOH mentioned by the client are education access and quality (did not graduate high school, low literacy level), economic stability (unemployed), health care access and quality (lack of medical insurance), and social and community context (effects on food choices).

   Ⓝ *NCLEX® Connection: Health Promotion and Maintenance, Health Promotion/Disease Prevention*

2. When generating solutions, the nurse should plan to include referrals to a social worker and case manager to work with the client for identification of community programs and other assistance programs. Resources the client may be interested in could include employment and education assistance, health insurance, food, utilities, and financial assistance for health care services. The nurse may refer the client to a pharmacist for consultation about lower-cost options for medications.

   Ⓝ *NCLEX® Connection: Alternations in Body Systems Illness Management*

3. When taking actions, the interprofessional health care team could assist with obtaining a home blood pressure cuff and scale. They could assist the client with finding pharmacies, community clinics, or community centers that have blood pressure monitors or scales the client can use free of charge.

   Ⓝ *NCLEX® Connection: Alternations in Body Systems Illness Management*

Application Exercises

1. A nurse is caring for a client who is transitioning to an oral diet following a partial laryngectomy. What are some actions the nurse should take to reduce the client's risk for aspiration?

2. A nurse is planning care for a client who has mechanical fixation of the jaw following a motorcycle crash. Which of the following actions should the nurse include in the plan of care? (Select all that apply.)
   - A. Thicken liquids to honey consistency.
   - B. Educate the client about the use of a nasogastric tube.
   - C. Assist the client to use a straw to drink liquids.
   - D. Ensure that the client receives ground meats.
   - E. Encourage intake of fluids between meals.

3. A nurse is caring for several clients in an extended care facility. Which of the following clients is the highest priority to observe during meals?
   - A. A client who has decreased vision
   - B. A client who has Parkinson's disease
   - C. A client who has poor dentition
   - D. A client who has anorexia

Active Learning Scenario

A nurse is planning care for an older adult who is at risk for malnutrition. The client is scheduled for discharge to their home where they live alone. The client reports that they have always been underweight, so they never paid attention to the nutrition values of foods. Use the ATI Active Learning Template: Basic Concept to complete this item to include the following sections.

UNDERLYING PRINCIPLES: Identify the client's barrier to nutrition.

NURSING INTERVENTIONS: Identify at least four interventions to address this client's barrier to nutrition and to promote healthy weight loss.

Application Exercises Key

1. When taking actions, the nurse should ensure that the client is sitting in an upright position before eating. The client should place a small amount, about ½ to 1 tsp of food in the mouth. The client should take a deep breath and bear down before swallowing the food. The client should flex the head toward the chest before swallowing. The client should cough or clear their throat after swallowing food. Other actions may include encouraging the client to rest before eating, ensuring that suction equipment is available, providing oral care before and after eating, and avoiding thin liquids.

   (N) *NCLEX® Connection: Reduction of Risk Potential, Potential for Alterations in Body Systems*

2. C, E. **CORRECT:** When generating solutions, the nurse should plan to assist the client to use a straw to drink liquids and should help the client determine where to insert the straw through the space between the jaws. The nurse should recognize that the client is only able to consume liquids and pureed foods and should plan to encourage supplemental and nutrient-rich liquids to maintain adequate hydration and nutrition.

   (N) *NCLEX® Connection: Basic Care and Comfort, Nutrition and Oral Hydration*

3. B. **CORRECT:** When prioritizing hypotheses using the airway, breathing, circulation approach to client care, the nurse determines that the client who has Parkinson's disease is at highest risk for aspiration, because the facial and pharyngeal muscles can become rigid, resulting in chewing and swallowing difficulties and is the highest priority to observe during meals.

   (N) *NCLEX® Connection: Reduction of Risk Potential, Potential for Alterations in Body Systems*

Active Learning Scenario Key

Using the ATI Active Learning Template: Basic Concept

UNDERLYING PRINCIPLES: The client's barrier to nutrition is lack of knowledge and misinformation about nutrition. This barrier must be acknowledged to promote adequate nutrition.

NURSING INTERVENTIONS
- Perform an assessment of dietary intake.
- Provide the client with information on healthy foods and nutrient values.
- Encourage the client to use dietary guidelines such as MyPlate.
- Assist the client in locating community resources that provide education and nutrition to support healthy nutrition.
- Consult social services to arrange home meal delivery.
- Advise the client to purchase frozen fruits and vegetables.
- Educate the client on how to read nutrition labels.
- Recommend drinking a supplement between meals.

(N) *NCLEX® Connection: Health Promotion and Maintenance, Health Promotion/Disease Prevention*

UNIT 3 ALTERATIONS IN NUTRITION

CHAPTER 12 *Malnutrition*

Malnutrition is caused by a lack of adequate nutrients or an imbalanced intake of nutrients and can be identified in clients who are underweight, overweight, or obese.

Malnutrition is a major cause of morbidity and mortality, decreased quality of life, and increased health care costs. Malnutrition can affect all organ systems, cause impaired cognition, and slow healing processes in clients who have had surgery. As a global health issue, poor nutrition increases risk for infectious diseases and conditions related to nutrient deficiencies, such as anemia. According to the World Health Organization (WHO), a greater number of people in the world live in countries in which the risk for death is greater from being overweight and obese than from being underweight.

NATIONAL HEALTH GOALS RELATED TO UNDERNUTRITION AND OVERNUTRITION ○EBP

Healthy People 2030, leading health indicators for nutrition and weight status, include:
- Increase the proportion of primary care physicians who regularly measure the body mass index of their adult clients.
- Increase the proportion of physician office visits made by adult clients who are obese that include counseling for education related to weight reduction, nutrition, or physical activity.
- Increase the proportion of adults who are at a healthy weight.
- Reduce household food insecurity and in so doing, reduce hunger. ○SDoH

Undernutrition

Additional information about specific vitamin and mineral deficiencies is available in the Sources of Nutrition chapter. Clients who have at least two of the following conditions meet diagnostic criteria for malnutrition, per the Academy of Nutrition and Dietetics:
- Inadequate intake of calories
- Loss of muscle mass
- Loss of subcutaneous fat
- Unintentional weight loss
- Decreased handgrip strength, indicating decreased functional status
- Weight loss masked by localized or generalized edema

Protein-energy malnutrition (PEM)

Also called protein-energy undernutrition
- Calorie deficit due to inadequate intake of protein, carbohydrates, and fat
  - May be starvation-related and is common in children affected by malnutrition, as well as older adults. **Starvation** is a complete lack of nutrients and does not involve inflammation.
  - **Marasmus**—Inadequate intake of calories and protein. Serum proteins may be within established ranges, but body fat and protein in the tissue are wasted.
  - **Kwashiorkor**—Lack of protein intake or intake of poor-quality protein in diet; calorie consumption may be adequate. Body weight may be within established ranges. Serum protein levels are low.

Chronic disease-related malnutrition

May occur in clients who have chronic disease processes
- Mild to moderate inflammation causes decreased appetite
- Underutilization of nutrients
- Examples:
  - Chronic alcohol use disorder is associated with poor diet.
    - Clients may have associated liver disorders.
    - Multivitamins and other oral nutritional supplements may be needed. Clients should use caution with any over-the-counter vitamins or other supplements that are not prescribed.
    - Thiamin absorption is impaired, and deficiency increases risk of alcoholic encephalopathies
    - If client has cirrhosis, deficiency of vitamins A, D, E, K is likely.
    - Ascites and abdominal pain from liver disease may affect appetite and comfort while eating.
  - COPD increases the work of breathing, which increases calories burned and increases risk for loss of muscle mass and strength
    - Poor appetite
    - Nausea
    - Abdominal bloating that leads to feeling of fullness
    - Dyspnea while eating

- HIV and AIDS increase the risk of wasting syndrome with loss of muscle mass
  - Diarrhea and malabsorption
  - Anorexia
  - Nausea
  - Difficulty swallowing if candida infection of throat or esophageal lesions are present
  - Medications may cause intolerance to fat
- Cystic fibrosis—decreased absorption of fat because of lack of pancreatic enzyme.
  - Work of breathing increases calorie expenditure
  - Abdominal distention, GERD may affect intake
  - Deficiency of vitamins, especially A, D, E, and K, is likely
- Chronic kidney disease increases risk of uremia and electrolyte imbalances
  - Protein and calorie needs are based on:
    - Height-to-weight ratio
    - Muscle tone
    - Serum albumin, hemoglobin, hematocrit
  - Protein restriction early in disease preserves kidney function
  - Protein needs may be different for clients who are undergoing hemodialysis or peritoneal dialysis

Acute disease-related or injury-related malnutrition

May occur in clients who have major infections, major traumas, or other critical conditions

- Clients may have been adequately nourished before illness or injury.
  - Severe inflammatory response during critical illness or injury causes decreased appetite and impaired digestion and absorption of nutrients. May require total parenteral nutrition (TPN) if gastrointestinal (GI) tract function is compromised.
- Malnutrition related to critical illnesses is associated with higher mortality rates, increased inpatient hospital days, and higher costs related hospitalization.
- Goals of nutritional support are to decrease morbidity from infections, total number of ventilator-dependent days, and length of stay in critical care units.
- Oral diet is preferred if possible. Enteral nutrition (EN) is preferred over parenteral nutrition (PN) if the GI tract is functioning.
- Fluid requirements must be individualized based on the presence of blood loss, diarrhea, vomiting, fever, and exudates.
- Indirect calorimetry (IC) provides the most accurate, predictive assessment of caloric needs.
  - Weight-based formula may be used if IC not available.
    - For clients who have BMI less than 30, 25 to 30 cal/kg/day, based on weight upon admission
    - For clients who have BMI 30 to 50, 11 to 14 cal/kg/day, based on weight upon admission
    - For clients who have BMI greater than 50, 22 to 25 cal/kg/day of ideal body weight

- For clients who have acute, critical illnesses, adequate protein intake may be more crucial than total calories.
  - For clients who have BMI less than 30, 1.2 to 2 g/kg/day of actual weight (may be higher for clients who have burns)
  - For clients who have BMI 30 to 40, 2 g/kg/day of ideal body weight
  - For clients who have BMI greater than 40, 2.5 g/kg/day of ideal body weight
- High doses of vitamins C and E and selenium, zinc, and copper are recommended.
- Examples:
  - Burns: caloric and nutrient needs increase because of increased metabolism and catabolism
    - Calorie-dense and protein-dense foods and oral supplements are sufficient if burns cover less than 20% of total body surface area (TBSA). Supplemental EN may be indicated if calorie and protein intake are less than 75% of estimated need for more than 3 days.
    - If client is unable to meet calorie needs with oral intake, initiation of EN (or PN if the GI tract is not functioning) within 4 to 6 hours of injury is associated with decreased risk for infection and improved function of the GI tract.
    - High metabolic rate may persist for years after injury.
  - Sepsis
    - Indirect calorimetry or weight-based equations should be used to calculate requirements for kcal/day.
    - Nutritional support through EN, or PN if the GI tract is not functioning, should be initiated as soon as possible.
  - Multi-trauma
    - Acute tissue injury and inflammation cause decreased prealbumin and albumin levels.
    - Head injuries
      - Client assumed to be in catabolic state
      - If skull fracture suspected or confirmed and client requires enteral feeding, oral feeding tube should be inserted instead of NG tube
    - After extubation, oral intake may be inadequate if diet is restrictive, if client is routinely NPO for tests and procedures, and if anorexia, nausea, or fatigue persist.

COMPLICATIONS OF UNDERNUTRITION

CARDIOVASCULAR AND RESPIRATORY
- Decreased cardiac output
- Decreased vital capacity

ENDOCRINE AND IMMUNOLOGIC
- Intolerance to cold
- Susceptibility to infectious diseases

GASTROINTESTINAL
- Vomiting
- Diarrhea
- Anorexia
- Malabsorption
- Impaired synthesis of proteins
- Weight loss

MUSCULOSKELETAL AND NEUROLOGIC
- Reduced activity tolerance
- Decrease in muscle mass
- Cachexia
- Impairments in functional ability
- Weakness

PSYCHIATRIC: Misuse of substances

INTEGUMENTARY
- Impaired wound healing
- Dermatitis
- Dryness and flakiness of skin

SOCIAL DETERMINANTS OF HEALTH THAT CONTRIBUTE TO MALNUTRITION Q SDoH

Additional information about social determinants of health that contribute to malnutrition is available in the **BARRIERS TO ADEQUATE NUTRITION CHAPTER.**
- Low income
- Lack of transportation
- Language barriers
- Lack of social support
- Lack of education about nutrition and food safety
- Low literacy level
- Contaminated soil and water

CULTURAL CONSIDERATIONS

It is important to recognize cultural considerations about the way food is prepared and presented. Malnutrition may result during a hospitalization or while residing in a community-living environment if the food provided does not meet cultural preferences.

OLDER ADULTS

Protein-energy malnutrition (PEM) is common in older adults who are in community-living environments or who are institutionalized.

Risk factors for malnutrition
Nutritional status and quality of life.
- Dental problems and difficulty swallowing
- Decreased senses of smell and taste
- Gastrointestinal manifestations, including constipation and dry mouth
- Musculoskeletal and neurological conditions
- Multiple medications increase likelihood of side effects and drug-nutrient interactions
- Challenges with purchasing and preparing food
- Losses of spouse or partner, friends, family members
- Social isolation

PATIENT-CENTERED CARE

The Joint Commission (TJC) set a standard for all clients to be screened within 24 hours of hospital admission. Treatment for malnutrition includes:
- Balanced, oral diet
- Liquid supplements
- Multivitamin supplements
- Correction of fluid and electrolyte imbalances
- Enteral feedings if client unable to consume adequate nutrients with oral intake
- Parenteral nutrition if client has GI tract impairments that interfere with absorption of nutrients

NURSING ACTIONS

Additional information about nutritional assessment and data collection is available in the Ingestion, Digestion, Absorption, and Metabolism and the Nutrition Assessment/Data Collection chapters.

Ongoing Assessment
- Document appetite, daily weights, and I&O. These activities may be delegated to AP with ongoing supervision.
- Monitor daily calorie count for some clients, for example, clients with burns
- Monitor laboratory studies:
  - Electrolytes and minerals
    - Decreased levels are associated with decreased nutrient intake.
    - Increased levels could be associated with high intake of one or more nutrients but lack of other nutrients in diet.
    - Hypernatremia could result from dehydration associated with malnutrition.
  - BUN—Negative nitrogen balance leads to decreased production of urea and decreased BUN.
  - Creatinine—Decreased creatinine level is associated with decreased muscle mass.
  - CBC—Anemias cause decreased red blood cell count (RBC), hematocrit (Hct), hemoglobin (Hg).
  - Liver function tests—May be indicated for clients who have substance use disorders or other conditions that involve liver damage.
  - Albumin and prealbumin
    - Because of shorter half-life than albumin, prealbumin is the best indicator of nutritional status—indicates what body has recently ingested, absorbed, digested, and metabolized.
    - Albumin and pre-albumin are synthesized in liver, so liver dysfunction causes decreased albumin and pre-albumin levels.
- Monitor manifestations of refeeding syndrome, which may occur with clients who are undernourished or malnourished when carbohydrates are reintroduced into the diet.
  - Replacement of carbohydrates stimulates insulin secretion and increases the need for nutrients involved in metabolism of carbohydrates.
  - Increased breakdown of carbohydrates leads to thiamin deficiency.
  - Electrolytes move into cells from the bloodstream.

- Supplementation of thiamin and electrolytes may be needed.
- If client is receiving EN or PN, rate may need to be slowed.
- Complications of refeeding syndrome include seizures, edema, heart failure, decreased serum levels of electrolytes, and hemolysis.

Interventions

- Requires collaboration with interprofessional team
  - Collaborate with provider and dietitian for ordering of diets that promote optimal nutrition.
  - Request consult from dietitian for clients with actual or potential for malnutrition.
  - Collaborate with dietitian and pharmacist for potential side effects of medications and medication-nutrient interactions that could affect absorption of nutrients.
  - If causes of malnutrition are related to inadequate resources, consult social worker or case manager.
  - Consult physical therapy and occupational therapy for functional issues.
- Educate clients about the importance of adequate nutrient intake.
- Counsel clients about drug-nutrient interactions that could affect absorption of nutrients.
- Assist clients with nutrient-dense food selection.
  - May require pureed, soft, or liquid diet if client has chewing or swallowing difficulties.
  - If the client is unable to meet nutrient requirement through oral intake, they may require supplemental enteral feedings or parental nutrition.

- In addition to choosing calorie-dense foods for meals and snacks, examples of other ways to increase calorie intake include these suggestions.
  - Add butter, mayonnaise, cream cheese, or olive oil to food.
  - Add honey to cereals.
  - Use gravy on meats and potatoes.
  - Add whipped cream to desserts and beverages.
- In addition to choosing protein-dense foods for meals snacks, examples of ways to increase protein intake include these suggestions.
  - Add cheese to vegetables, sandwiches, and salads.
  - Add peanut butter to cereal or dip fruit into peanut butter.
  - Add nuts to cereals, desserts, and salads.
  - Mix fruit with yogurt.
  - Use milk instead of water in recipes.

NURSING ACTIONS TO PROMOTE OPTIMAL INTAKE

Environment

- Provide pain management interventions before meals.
- Decrease strong odors. For example, remove lids from foods before placing in front of client.
- Eliminate environmental distractions as much as possible.
- Clear eating area of urinals, bedpans, and emesis basins.

12.1 Case Study

Scenario introduction
A nurse on the medical-surgical unit is caring for a client who is at risk for malnutrition.

Scene 1
The client is lying in bed when the nurse enters the room. The client has not eaten anything from the meal tray on the overbed table beside the bed.

Client: I don't feel much like eating. My leg really hurts right now.

Nurse: How would you rate your pain on a scale from 0 to 10?

Client: It's at an 8.

Nurse: Would you like to have your pain medication?

Client: Yes, please. I'm really uncomfortable.

Scene 2
The nurse returns to the client's room.

Nurse: It has been about 20 minutes since you had your pain medication. How do you rate your pain now?

Client: It's at about a 5, so it's better.

Nurse: Do you want to try to eat now?

Client: I don't have much of an appetite here. Even the smell of food makes me lose my appetite.

Nurse: I will reheat your food, then let's see how we can make you more comfortable so you can eat.

Scenario conclusion
The nurse returns to the room with the tray.

Case study exercises

1. The nurse provided pain management for the client and reheated food on the meal tray that is no longer warm. What other actions can the nurse implement for this client to promote intake of this meal?

2. Which is the reason the nurse would monitor albumin levels for this client?
   A. Albumin levels may indicate severity of disease.
   B. Albumin is the most reliable indicator of protein malnutrition.
   C. Increased albumin levels indicate increased inflammation.
   D. Increased albumin levels indicate fluid overload.

Comfort

- Provide opportunity for hygiene activities before meals; for example, toileting, oral care, hand hygiene.
- Assist client to a sitting position, in a chair if possible.
- Encourage client to use hearing aids, eyeglasses, and other assistive devices during meals.

Function

- Eliminate or minimize non-urgent care activities and procedures during mealtimes.
- Ensure appropriate temperature of foods and fluids.
- Encourage client to feed themselves as much as possible.
- Assist client to open packages and cut food if needed.
- Assist client with feeding if needed. Allow adequate time for client to chew and swallow.
- Observe and document intake.

Obesity

- Obesity is a chronic condition caused by calorie intake in excess of energy expenditure. It can be affected by numerous factors (culture, metabolism, environment, socioeconomics, individual behaviors). Q**SDoH**
- Obesity might be linked to protective measures within the body to prevent weight loss during calorie restriction, which cause it to secrete hormones that stimulate the appetite to maintain a specific weight. As weight increases, the body accepts a higher weight as the expected weight and seeks to maintain it.

ASSESSMENT

Additional information about nutritional assessment and data collection is available in the Ingestion, Digestion, Absorption, and Metabolism and the Nutrition Assessment/Data Collection chapters.

RISK FACTORS

- Genetic predisposition
- Hormones (leptin, ghrelin)
- Behavioral factors (sedentary lifestyle, diet choices)

EXPECTED FINDINGS

Clients report of depression, low self-esteem, avoidance of health-related appointments, and no desire to exercise because of feeling stigmatized by their excessive weight.

BODY MASS INDEX

- Overweight: 25 to 29.9
- Obesity: 30 or greater

WAIST CIRCUMFERENCE

- Females: greater than 88.9 cm (35 in)
- Males: greater than 101.6 cm (40 in)

WAIST-TO-HIP RATIO (WHR)

- Measurement of difference between peripheral lower body obesity and central obesity
- Can be used as a predictor of coronary artery disease
- Indicates excess fat at the waist and abdomen
  - Males: 0.95 or greater
  - Females: 0.8 or greater

LABORATORY TESTS

- Screening to evaluate for cardiovascular disease, diabetes mellitus, fatty liver disease, or thyroid disorders
- Total cholesterol
- Triglycerides
- Fasting blood glucose
- Glycosylated hemoglobin
- Aspartate aminotransferase (AST)
- Alanine aminotransferase (ALT)

COMPLICATIONS OF OBESITY

CARDIOVASCULAR AND RESPIRATORY

- Coronary artery disease (CAD)
- Hypertension
- Hyperlipidemia
- Asthma
- Obstructive sleep apnea

ENDOCRINE AND IMMUNOLOGIC

- Prediabetes
- Type 2 diabetes mellitus
- Nonalcoholic fatty liver disease
- Susceptibility to infection from poor wound healing
- Increased risk of certain cancers:
  - Breast
  - Colon
  - Endometrial
  - Esophageal
  - Kidney
  - Pancreatic

GASTROINTESTINAL

- Gastroesophageal reflux disease (GERD)
- Cholelithiasis

MUSCULOSKELETAL AND NEUROLOGIC

- Osteoarthritis
- Stroke

PSYCHIATRIC AND PSYCHOLOGICAL

- Binge-eating
- Anxiety
- Depression

REPRODUCTIVE AND GENITOURINARY

- Polycystic ovary syndrome
- Hypogonadism
- Urinary stress incontinence

Obesity also increases the risk for perioperative complications and complications during pregnancy, labor, and birth.

PATIENT-CENTERED CARE

REDUCED CALORIE DIET

- Healthy eating plans include DASH, Mediterranean, vegetarian Q**EBP**
- Decrease of 500 to 750 kcal/day
- Very low–calorie diets (less than 800 kcal/day are only for limited use, such as weight reduction before bariatric surgery, and must be under medical supervision).

PHYSICAL ACTIVITY

- Decrease time spent in sedentary activities.
- Increase aerobic and resistance exercises.

BEHAVIOR MODIFICATION STRATEGIES:

- Goal setting
- Avoidance of triggers
- In-person or remote support group meetings
- Behavior change contract
- Stress management activities
- Motivational interviewing

MEDICATIONS

- Approved by the FDA for clients who have a BMI of 30 or greater and no complications, or for clients who have a BMI of 27 or greater and at least one complication.
- Clients who do not lose weight during weight loss programs can benefit from pharmacological therapy.
- Anorectic medications suppress appetite and reduce food intake. When combined with an exercise program, they can result in weight loss.

INTERPROFESSIONAL CARE

The care team can include a health care provider, nursing team, dietitian, social worker, surgeon, and mental health therapist or counselor.

NURSING CARE
Maintain low-Fowler's position to maximize chest expansion.

CLIENT EDUCATION: Follow the prescribed diet from the provider or dietitian to prevent complications of obesity.

SURGICAL INTERVENTIONS

Bariatric surgery

This is considered the most effective treatment for managing obesity and related conditions. Benefits include reduction of diabetes mellitus, hypertension, dyslipidemia, and mortality rates as well as improved quality of life.

Clients who are candidates for bariatric surgery:
- Clients with BMI of 40 or greater and no complications from obesity
- Clients with BMI of 35 or greater and one or more obesity related complications
- Clients with BMI between 30 and 34.9 who have type 2 diabetes that is not well controlled with diet, physical activity, and medications

Bariatric surgery works best in combination with diet and lifestyle changes. Nutritional counseling is essential. Protein intake of 60 g/day or more is required to prevent protein-calorie malnutrition.

Common nutritional deficiencies after bariatric surgeries include iron, calcium, thiamin, vitamin B_{12}, and vitamin D.
- Malabsorption of iron—oral or parental iron supplementation may be needed.
- Malabsorption of vitamin B_{12}—oral supplementation or monthly vitamin B_{12} injections may be needed.

CLIENT EDUCATION: Dramatic changes in food intake and regular physical activity will be necessary for successful long-term weight control.

Adjustable gastric banding restricts stomach capacity to 15 to 30 mL with an inflatable band that encircles the uppermost portion of the stomach, similar to a belt to create an outlet that can be adjusted as needed.

CLIENT EDUCATION

- Diet will gradually increase from liquids to pureed to soft foods.
- Chew foods thoroughly, slowly, and in small amounts.

Roux-en-Y gastric bypass: Ingested food bypasses the majority of the stomach, the duodenum, and a small portion of the proximal jejunum. Weight loss is achieved through gastric restriction and malabsorption.
- Possible postoperative complications include anastomotic leaks, GI bleeding, stomal stenosis, and dumping syndrome.
- Micronutrient deficiencies are common long term.

Sleeve gastrectomy is a procedure in which a longitudinal portion of the stomach is removed to create a "sleeve" effect. This 80% reduction of stomach capacity leads to an increase in hormones that promote satiety.

1. A nurse is caring for multiple clients who are malnourished. The nurse should identify that which of the following client conditions are associated with severe inflammation that can lead to malnutrition? (Select all that apply.)

   A. Sepsis

   B. Cystic fibrosis

   C. Starvation

   D. Chronic kidney disease

   E. Third-degree burns

   F. Chronic alcohol use disorder

   G. AIDS

2. A nurse in a bariatric clinic is caring for a group of clients who are being evaluated for bariatric surgery. Which of the following clients does the nurse recognize as the most appropriate candidate for education about bariatric surgery?

   A. Client who has BMI of 27 and type 2 diabetes

   B. Client who has BMI of 34 and asthma

   C. Client who has BMI of 35 and osteoarthritis

   D. Client who has BMI of 38 and no obesity-related complications

3. A nurse is preparing a presentation about complications of undernutrition and obesity. Sort the characteristics that are more likely associated with undernutrition and those more likely associated with obesity.

   A. Intolerance to cold

   B. Increased risk of colon cancer

   C. Sleep apnea

   D. Stress urinary incontinence

   E. Diarrhea

A nurse is providing dietary teaching for a client who requests assistance for weight loss. The client states, "I've tried several fad diets that completely eliminate certain foods like carbohydrates or fats but they don't work for me." Use the ATI Active Learning Template: Basic Concept to complete this item to include the following sections.

UNDERLYING PRINCIPLES: Identify the client's barrier to nutrition.

NURSING INTERVENTIONS: Identify at least four interventions to address this client's barrier to nutrition and to promote healthy weight loss.

Application Exercises Key

1. A, E. **CORRECT:** When analyzing cues, the nurse should recognize that sepsis and third-degree burns are client conditions that are associated with severe inflammation that can lead to malnutrition. Severe inflammation from critical illness or injury causes decreased appetite and impaired digestion and absorption of nutrients.

   Ⓝ *NCLEX® Connection: Basic Care and Comfort, Nutrition and Oral Hydration*

2. C. **CORRECT:** When recognizing cues, the nurse identifies the client who has a BMI of 35 and osteoarthritis as the most appropriate candidate for bariatric surgery. A client who has a BMI of 35 or greater and one or more comorbid conditions or complications that may be remedied with weight loss is a candidate for bariatric surgery.

   Ⓝ *NCLEX® Connection: Reduction of Risk Potential, Therapeutic Procedures*

3. **UNDERNUTRITION**: A, E ; **OBESITY**: B, C, D,

   When generating solutions, the nurse identifies intolerance to cold and diarrhea as manifestations of undernutrition. Diminished fat stores under the skin affect insulation against the cold. Diarrhea may be caused or worsened by lack of lactase, as well as the increased risk for infection of the intestinal tract. The nurse identifies increased risk of colon cancer, obstructive sleep apnea, and stress urinary incontinence as conditions that are associated with obesity. Evidence indicates an association between obesity and the development of colon cancer. Fat deposits in the neck contribute to narrowing of the airway and increase risks for obstructive sleep apnea. Management of stress urinary incontinence for clients who have obesity includes weight reduction.

   Ⓝ *NCLEX® Connection: Basic Care and Comfort, Nutrition and Oral Hydration*

Active Learning Scenario Key

Using the ATI Active Learning Template: Basic Concepts

UNDERLYING PRINCIPLES: The client's barrier to nutrition is lack of knowledge and misinformation about nutrition. This barrier must be acknowledged to promote adequate nutrition.

NURSING INTERVENTIONS
- Encourage the client to use dietary guidelines such as MyPlate.
- Assist the client in locating community resources that provide education and nutrition to support healthy nutrition and weight loss.
- Advise the client that fad diets are generally unhealthy and often include false advertising.
- Perform an assessment of dietary intake.
- Encourage the client to keep a journal of dietary intake.
- Provide the client with information on healthy foods and portion sizes.

Ⓝ *NCLEX® Connection: Health Promotion and Maintenance, Health Promotion/Disease Prevention*

Case Study Exercises Key

1. When taking actions, the nurse should eliminate strong odors that increase the likelihood of nausea by removing lids from plates, bowls, and cups before placing the tray in front of the client. The nurse should assist the client to a sitting position to facilitate comfort and swallowing. The nurse should identify the need for and provide the client with their glasses, hearing aids, dentures, and other assistive devices to promote independence. The nurse should encourage toileting, hand hygiene, and oral hygiene before the meal to facilitate comfort and the sense of taste.

2. **A:** When analyzing cues, the nurse should recognize that albumin levels decrease in the presence of inflammation and are a good indicator of the progression and severity of disease.

CHAPTER 13 *Cardiovascular and Hematologic Disorders*

Nurses must have an awareness of nutritional needs for clients who have cardiovascular and hematologic disorders. It is important to explore dietary needs with the client and recommend modifications related to the disease process.

In the United States, heart disease is the leading cause of death. Therefore, understanding the role of primary and secondary prevention is essential to successful prevention and treatment.

ASSESSMENT/DATA COLLECTION

Coronary heart disease

Hypercholesterolemia leads to atherosclerosis, a process of damage and cholesterol deposits on the blood vessels of the heart. Atherosclerosis is the cause of many cardiovascular disease complications (myocardial infarction, kidney failure, ischemic strokes).

- High-density lipoprotein (HDL) cholesterol is "good" cholesterol because it removes cholesterol from the body tissue and takes it to the liver. Levels greater than or equal to 60 mg/dL for males and 70 mg/dL or greater for females provide some protection against heart disease.
- Low-density lipoprotein (LDL) cholesterol is "bad" cholesterol because it transports cholesterol out of the liver and into the circulatory system, where it can form plaques on the coronary artery walls. The optimal range for LDL is less than 130 mg/dL.
- Optimal total cholesterol level is less than 200 mg/dL. Q EBP

RISK FACTORS

- **NON-MODIFIABLE:** increasing age, male sex, family history of early CHD
- **MODIFIABLE:** high LDL cholesterol, low HDL cholesterol, consuming a diet high in saturated fat, hypertension, diabetes mellitus, metabolic syndrome, obesity, sedentary lifestyle, nicotine use disorder

Metabolic syndrome

The presence of three of the five following risk factors.
- Abdominal obesity
  - **MALES:** greater than or equal to 40-inch waist
  - **FEMALES:** greater than or equal to 35-inch waist
  - For Asian and non-European clients who have lived predominantly outside the U.S., use population- or country-specific definitions.

- Triglycerides greater than or equal to 150 mg/dL or taking medications to treat high triglyceride levels
- Low HDL or taking medications to lower HDL–C
  - **MALES:** less than or equal to 40 mg/dL
  - **FEMALES:** less than or equal to 50 mg/dL
- Increased blood pressure or taking an antihypertensive medication
  - Systolic greater than or equal to 130 mm/Hg
  - Diastolic greater than or equal to 80 mm/Hg
- Fasting blood glucose greater than or equal to 100 mg/dL or taking medication to control blood glucose levels

ANEMIAS

Iron deficiency anemia

RISK FACTORS

- Blood loss, deficient iron intake from diet, alcohol use disorder, malabsorption syndromes, gastrectomy
- Metabolic increase caused by pregnancy, adolescence, infection

MANIFESTATIONS

- Fatigue
- Lethargy
- Pallor of nail beds
- Intolerance to cold
- Headache
- Tachycardia

! Children who have low iron intake can experience short attention spans and display poor intellectual performance before anemia begins.

Vitamin B$_{12}$ deficiency anemia (macrocytic)

RISK FACTORS: Lack of meat or dairy consumption, small bowel resection, chronic diarrhea, diverticula, tapeworm, excess of intestinal bacteria

MANIFESTATIONS

- Pallor
- Jaundice
- Weakness
- Fatigue

GASTROINTESTINAL FINDINGS

- Glossitis (inflamed tongue)
- Anorexia
- Indigestion
- Weight loss

NEUROLOGIC FINDINGS

- Decreased concentration
- Paresthesia (numbness) of hands and feet
- Decreased proprioception (sense of body position)
- Poor muscle coordination
- Increasing irritability
- Delirium

Folic acid deficiency anemia

RISK FACTORS: Poor nutritional intake of foods containing folic acid (green leafy vegetables, citrus fruits, dried bean, nuts), malabsorption syndromes (Crohn's disease), certain medications (anticonvulsants and oral contraceptives)

MANIFESTATIONS
- Fatigue
- Pallor
- Glossitis
- Irritability
- Diarrhea

> Findings of folic acid deficiency anemia mimic those for vitamin B_{12} deficiency anemia except for the neurologic manifestations.

NUTRITIONAL GUIDELINES AND NURSING INTERVENTIONS

Coronary heart disease

PREVENTATIVE NUTRITION
- Consuming a diet that is limited in trans fats, saturated fats, and cholesterol can reduce the risk of developing CHD. The Therapeutic Lifestyle Change (TLC) diet is designed to be a user-friendly eating guide to encourage dietary changes.
- Daily cholesterol intake should be less than 200 mg.
- Conservative use of red wine can reduce the risk of developing CHD.
- Increasing fiber and carbohydrate intake, avoiding saturated fat, and decreasing red meat consumption can decrease the risk for developing CHD.
- Increased intake of omega-3 fatty acids found in fish, flaxseed, soybeans, canola, and walnuts reduces the risk of coronary artery disease.
- Homocysteine is an amino acid. Elevated homocysteine levels can increase the risk of developing CHD. Deficiencies in folate and vitamins B_6 and B_{12} increase homocysteine levels.

THERAPEUTIC NUTRITION
- Secondary prevention efforts for CHD are focused on lifestyle changes that lower LDL. These include a diet low in cholesterol and saturated fats, a diet high in fiber, exercise and weight management, and cessation of nicotine use.
- Daily cholesterol intake should be less than 200 mg/day. Saturated fat should be limited to less than 7% of daily caloric intake.
- To lower cholesterol and saturated fats, instruct the client to do the following.
  - Trim visible fat from meats.
  - Limit red meats and choose lean meats (turkey, chicken).
  - Remove the skin from meats.
  - Broil, bake, grill, or steam foods. Avoid frying foods.
  - Use low-fat or nonfat milk, cheese, and yogurt.
  - Use spices in place of butter or salt to season foods.

- Use liquid oils (olive or canola) in place of oils that are high in saturated fat (lard, butter).
  - Avoid trans-fat, which increases LDL. Partially hydrogenated products contain trans-fat.
  - Increase consumption of oily fish (tuna, salmon, herring). Q^{SDoH}
  - Read labels.
- Encourage the client to consume a high-fiber diet.
  - Soluble fiber lowers LDL.
  - Oats, beans, fruits, vegetables, whole grains, barley, and flaxseed are good sources of fiber.
- Encourage the client to exercise.
  - Instruct the client regarding practical methods for increasing physical activity. (Encourage the client to take the stairs rather than the elevator.)
  - Provide the client with references for local exercise facilities.
- Instruct the client to stop all use of tobacco products.
- The recommended lifestyle changes represent a significant change for many clients. Q^{PCC}
  - Provide support to the client and family.
  - Encourage the client's family to participate in the changes to ease the transition for the client.
  - Explain why the diet is important.
  - Aid the client in developing a diet that is complementary to personal food preferences and lifestyle. A food diary can be helpful.
  - Instruct the client that occasional deviations from the diet are reasonable.
  - Collaborate with the interprofessional team to connect clients who live in food desserts or who face financial challenges with resources for nutritious food options. Q^{TC}

Hypertension

- Hypertension is a significant risk factor for developing CHD, myocardial infarction, kidney disease, and stroke.
- Hypertension is a sustained elevation in blood pressure greater than or equal to 130/80 mm Hg.

RISK FACTORS FOR PRIMARY HYPERTENSION: family history, hyperlipidemia, smoking, obesity, physical inactivity, high sodium intake, low potassium intake, excessive alcohol consumption, stress, and aging. African-American people have the highest prevalence of hypertension. A client's risk of hypertension increases after menopause.

THERAPEUTIC NUTRITION
- The Dietary Approaches to Stopping Hypertension (DASH) diet is a low-sodium, high-potassium, high-calcium diet that has proven to lower blood pressure (systolic and diastolic) and cholesterol.
  - Decrease sodium intake (initially a daily intake of less than 2,300 mg is recommended and should gradually be decreased to 1,500 mg for maximum benefit).
  - Foods high in sodium include canned soups and sauces, potato chips, pretzels, smoked meats, seasonings, and processed foods.
  - Include low-fat dairy products to promote calcium intake.
  - Include fruits and vegetables rich in potassium (apricots, bananas, tomatoes, potatoes).

- Limit alcohol intake.
- Encourage the client to read labels and educate the client about appropriate food choices.
- Other lifestyle changes include exercising, weight loss, and smoking cessation.

Heart failure

Heart failure is characterized by the inability of the heart to maintain adequate blood flow throughout the circulatory system. It results in excess sodium and fluid retention, and edema.

RISK FACTORS: CHD, arrhythmias, previous MI, valve disorders, hypertension, obesity, diabetes, metabolic syndrome

THERAPEUTIC NUTRITION
- Reduce sodium intake to less than 3,000 mg per day for mild-to-moderate heart failure and less than 2,000 mg/day for severe heart failure.
- Monitor fluid intake (and possibly restrict 2 L/day).
- Increase protein intake to 1.12 g/kg.
- Use small, frequent meals that are soft, easy-to-chew foods.

Myocardial infarction

- A myocardial infarction (MI) occurs when there is an inadequate supply of oxygen to the myocardium.
- After an MI, it is necessary to reduce the myocardial oxygen demands related to metabolic activity.
- Risk factors are the same as for CHD.

THERAPEUTIC NUTRITION
- A liquid diet is best for the first 24 hr after the infarction.
- Caffeine should be avoided because it stimulates the heart and increases heart rate.
- Small, frequent meals are indicated.
- Counsel the client about recommendations for a heart-healthy diet.

Anemia

Anemia results from either a reduction in the number of red blood cells (RBCs) or in hemoglobin, the oxygen-carrying component of blood. Anemia can result from a decrease in RBC production, an increase in RBC destruction, or a loss of blood.
- The body requires iron, vitamin B_{12}, and folic acid to produce red blood cells.
- Iron deficiency anemia is the most common nutritional disorder in the world. It affects approximately 10% of the U.S. population, especially older infants, toddlers, adolescent females, and pregnant clients.
- From childhood until adolescence, iron intake tends to be marginal.
- Pernicious anemia is the most common form of vitamin B_{12} deficiency. It is caused by lack of intrinsic factor, a protein that helps the body absorb vitamin B_{12}.

SOURCES OF IRON
- Red meat
- Fish
- Poultry
- Tofu
- Dried peas and beans
- Whole grains
- Dried fruit
- Iron-fortified foods
  - Infant formula (alternative or supplement to breastfeeding)
  - Infant cereal (usually the first food introduced to infants)
  - Ready-to-eat cereals

VITAMIN C: Facilitates the absorption of iron (promote consumption).

! Medicinal iron toxicity is the leading cause of accidental poisoning in small children and can lead to acute iron toxicity. Qs

NATURAL SOURCES OF VITAMIN B_{12}
- Fish
- Meat
- Poultry
- Eggs
- Milk

People older than 50 years are urged to consume most of their vitamin B_{12} requirement from supplements or fortified food.

People who follow a vegan diet need supplemental B_{12}.

FOLIC ACID SOURCES
- Green leafy vegetables
- Dried peas and beans
- Seeds
- Orange juice
- Cereals and breads fortified with folic acid

If the client is unable to obtain an adequate supply of folic acid, supplementation can be necessary.

Active Learning Scenario

A nurse is providing teaching to a client who has hypertension. What should the nurse include in the teaching? Use the ATI Active Learning Template: System Disorder to complete this item to include the following sections.

ALTERATION IN HEALTH (DIAGNOSIS)

CLIENT EDUCATION: Describe the Dietary Approaches to Stopping Hypertension (DASH) diet and four nutrition teaching points to include.

Application Exercises

1. A nurse is reviewing a client health record that includes a report of abdominal obesity and laboratory findings of elevated blood glucose and elevated triglycerides. The nurse should identify that these findings meet the criteria of which of the following conditions?

   A. Anemia

   B. Metabolic syndrome

   C. Heart failure

   D. Hypertension

2. A community health nurse is assessing a client who reports numbness of the hands and feet for the past 2 weeks. The nurse should identify this finding as a manifestation of which of the following nutritional deficiencies?

   A. Folic acid

   B. Potassium

   C. Vitamin B$_{12}$

   D. Iron

3. A nurse is teaching a client about high-fiber foods that can assist in lowering LDL. Which of the following foods should the nurse include? (Select all that apply.)

   A. Beans

   B. Cheese

   C. Whole grains

   D. Broccoli

   E. Yogurt

4. A nurse is teaching a client about dietary recommendations to lower high blood pressure. Which of the following statements by the client indicates understanding?

   A. "My daily sodium consumption should be 3,000 milligrams."

   B. "I should consume foods low in potassium."

   C. "My limit is three cigarettes a day."

   D. "I should consume low-fat dairy products."

5. A nurse is providing teaching to a client who has vitamin B$_{12}$ deficiency. Which of the following foods should the nurse instruct the client to consume? (Select all that apply.)

   A. Meat

   B. Flaxseed

   C. Beans

   D. Eggs

   E. Milk

Application Exercises Key

1. B. **CORRECT:** The nurse should analyze cues from the client's history and determine that weight gain in the abdomen, elevated blood glucose, and elevated triglycerides are manifestations associated with metabolic syndrome.

   Ⓝ *NCLEX® Connection: Basic Care and Comfort, Nutrition and Oral Hydration*

2. C. **CORRECT:** The nurse should analyze the cues from the client's assessment and identify that numbness of the hands and feet are manifestations associated with vitamin B$_{12}$ deficiency.

   Ⓝ *NCLEX® Connection: Basic Care and Comfort, Nutrition and Oral Hydration*

3. A, C, D. **CORRECT:** When taking actions and teaching a client about foods that can assist with lowering LDL cholesterol, the nurse should include that beans are high in fiber as well as whole grains and broccoli.

   Ⓝ *NCLEX® Connection: Basic Care and Comfort, Nutrition and Oral Hydration*

4. D. **CORRECT:** When evaluation outcomes of client teaching about dietary recommendations to lower blood pressure, the nurse should identify client understanding when the client states they should consume low-fat dairy products. Low-fat dairy products should be encouraged, as they promote calcium intake and assist with lowering systolic and diastolic blood pressures as well as cholesterol.

   Ⓝ *NCLEX® Connection: Basic Care and Comfort, Nutrition and Oral Hydration*

5. A, D, E. **CORRECT:** When taking actions and teaching a client about foods that are high in vitamin B$_{12}$, the nurse should recommend meat, eggs, and milk to the client.

   Ⓝ *NCLEX® Connection: Basic Care and Comfort, Nutrition and Oral Hydration*

Active Learning Scenario Key

Using the ATI Active Learning Template: System Disorder

ALTERATION IN HEALTH (DIAGNOSIS): Hypertension is a sustained elevation in blood pressure greater than or equal to 140/90 mm Hg in clients less than age 60 and 150/90 mm Hg in those older than 60.

CLIENT EDUCATION

- The DASH diet is a low-sodium, high-potassium, high-calcium diet that has been proven to lower blood pressure and cholesterol.
- Lower sodium intake (daily intake of less than 2,300 mg) is recommended.
- Foods high in sodium include canned soups and sauces, potato chips, pretzels, smoked meats, seasonings, and processed foods.
- Include low-fat dairy products to promote calcium intake.
- Include fruits and vegetables rich in potassium (apricots, bananas, tomatoes, potatoes).
- Limit alcohol intake.

Ⓝ *NCLEX® Connection: Physiological Adaptation, Illness Management*

UNIT 3   ALTERATIONS IN NUTRITION

CHAPTER 14 *Gastrointestinal Disorders*

Nurses need to have an awareness of nutritional needs for clients who have gastrointestinal (GI) disorders. It is important to explore dietary needs with the client and recommend modifications in relationship to the disease process. Understanding the role of primary and secondary prevention is essential to successful treatment.

Nutrition therapy for gastrointestinal disorders is generally aimed at minimizing or preventing manifestations. In some conditions (celiac disease), nutrition is the only treatment. For some GI disorders, nutrition therapy is the foundation of treatment.

ASSESSMENT/DATA COLLECTION

- Determine whether the client is experiencing any of the following.
  - Difficulty chewing or swallowing
  - Nausea, vomiting, or diarrhea
  - Bloating, excessive flatus, occult blood, steatorrhea, abdominal pain or cramping, abdominal distention, pale, sticky bowel movements
  - Changes in weight, eating patterns, or bowel habits
- Determine whether the client uses the following.
  - Tobacco
  - Alcohol
  - Caffeine
  - Over-the-counter medications to treat GI conditions (many can have GI complications or be contraindicated with GI conditions)
  - Nutritional supplements
  - Herbal supplements for GI conditions or other problems (some clients do not consider them to be medications, so they do not mention them to the provider)

NUTRITIONAL GUIDELINES AND NURSING INTERVENTIONS

General gastrointestinal considerations

- Monitor gastrointestinal parameters.
  - Weight and weight changes
  - Laboratory values
  - Elimination patterns
  - I&O
- Low-fiber diets avoid foods that are high in residue content (whole-grain breads and cereals, raw fruits and vegetables).
  - Diets low in fiber reduce the frequency and volume of fecal output and slow transit time of food through the digestive tract.
  - Low-fiber diets are used short-term for clients who have diarrhea or malabsorption syndromes.
- High-fiber diets focus on foods containing more than 5 g of fiber per serving. A diet high in fiber helps:
  - Increase stool bulk.
  - Stimulate peristalsis.
  - Prevent constipation.
  - Protect against colon cancer.

Nausea and vomiting

- Potential causes of nausea and vomiting include decreased gastric acid secretion; decreased gastrointestinal motility; allergy to food(s); bacterial or viral infection; increased intracranial pressure; liver, pancreatic, and gall bladder disorders; and adverse effects of some medications.
- The underlying cause of nausea and vomiting should be investigated. Assessing the appearance of the emesis will aid in diagnosis and treatment (coffee-ground emesis indicates the presence of blood; pale green indicates bile).
- Once manifestations subside, begin with clear liquids followed by full liquids, and advance the diet as tolerated.
- Easy-to-digest, low-fat carbohydrate foods (crackers, toast, oatmeal, pretzels, plain bread, bland fruit) are usually well-tolerated.

NURSING ACTIONS
- Promote good oral hygiene with tooth brushing, mouth swabs, mouthwash, and ice chips.
- Elevate the head of the bed.
- Serve foods at room temperature or chilled.

CLIENT EDUCATION
- Avoid hot and spicy foods.
- Avoid liquids with meals, as they promote a feeling of fullness.
- Avoid high-fat foods if they contribute to nausea because they are difficult to digest.

Anorexia

- Anorexia is defined as a lack of appetite. It is a common finding for numerous physical conditions and is an adverse effect of certain medications. It is not the same as anorexia nervosa.
- Anorexia can lead to decreased nutritional intake and subsequent protein and calorie deficits.

NURSING ACTIONS

- Decrease stress at mealtimes.
- Collect data regarding adverse effects of medications.
- Administer medications to stimulate appetite.
- Assess and modify environment for unpleasant odors.
- Remove items that cause a decrease in appetite (soiled linens, garbage, emesis basins, bedpans, used tissues, clutter).
- Assess and manage anxiety and depression.
- Provide small, frequent meals and avoid high-fat foods to help maximize intake. Beverages should be held at least 30 min before and after meals to prevent the client from feeling full before adequate intake of calories from food.
- Provide liquid supplements between meals to improve protein and calorie intake.
- Ensure that meals appear appealing. Serve larger meals early in the day.
- Season food according to taste, for decreased ability to taste, enhance foods with tart (orange juice, lemon juice) or strong seasonings (basil, oregano).
- Assess for changes in bowel status (increased gastric emptying, constipation, diarrhea).
- Position to increase gastric motility.
- Provide mouth care before and after meals.

Constipation

- Clients who have constipation have difficult or infrequent passage of stools, which can be hard and dry.
- Causes include irregular bowel habits, psychogenic factors, inactivity, chronic laxative use, obstruction, medications, GI disorders (irritable bowel syndrome [IBS]), pregnancy, or secondary to genital/rectal trauma (sexual abuse or childbirth), and inadequate consumption of fiber and fluid.
- Encourage exercise and a diet high in fiber (25 g/day for females and 38 g/day for males) and promote adequate fluid intake to help alleviate constipation.
- If caused by medication, a change in the medication might be necessary.

NURSING ACTIONS

- Determine onset and duration of past and present elimination patterns, what is normal for the client, activity levels, occupation, dietary intake, and stress levels.
- Collect data about past medical and surgical history, medication use (OTC, herbal supplements, laxatives, enemas, and prescriptions), presence of rectal pressure or fullness, and abdominal pain.
- Encourage client to gradually increase daily intake of fiber.

CLIENT EDUCATION

- Increase fluid intake to 64 oz/day unless contraindicated.
- An increase in fiber intake is the preferred treatment for constipation. Avoid chronic use of laxatives.

Diarrhea

- Diarrhea can cause significant losses of potassium, sodium, and fluid, as well as nutritional complications.
- Common causes of diarrhea include emotional and physical stress, gastrointestinal disorders, malabsorption disorders, infections, and certain medications.
- Low-fiber diets might be recommended on a short-term basis to decrease bowel stimulation.
- Nutrition therapy varies with the severity and duration of diarrhea. A liberal fluid intake to replace losses is needed.

Dysphagia

- Dysphagia is an alteration in the client's ability to swallow.
- Causes include obstruction, inflammation, and certain neurologic disorders.
- Modifying the texture of foods and the consistency of liquids can enable the client to achieve proper nutrition.
- Dry mouth can contribute to dysphagia. Evaluate medications being taken to determine if this is a potential adverse effect.
- Clients who have dysphagia should be referred to a speech therapist for evaluation.
- Dietary modifications are based on the specific swallowing limitations experienced by the client.
- Nutritional supplements are beneficial if nutritional intake is deemed inadequate.

NURSING ACTIONS

- Clients who have dysphagia are at an increased risk of aspiration. Place the client in an upright or high-Fowler's position to facilitate swallowing. **Qs**
- Provide oral care prior to eating to enhance the client's sense of taste.
- Allow adequate time for eating, use adaptive eating devices, and encourage small bites and thorough chewing.

CLIENT EDUCATION

- Pills should be taken with at least 8 oz of fluid (can be thickened) to prevent medication from remaining in the esophagus.
- Avoid thin liquids and sticky foods.

Dumping syndrome

Normally, the stomach controls the rate in which nutrients enter the small intestine. When a portion of the stomach is surgically removed, the contents of the stomach are rapidly emptied into the small intestine, causing dumping syndrome.

- Early manifestations typically occur 10 to 20 min after eating. Early manifestations include a sensation of fullness, abdominal cramping, nausea, diarrhea, and vasomotor manifestations (faintness, syncope, diaphoresis, tachycardia, hypotension, flushing).
- Late manifestations occur 1 to 3 hr after eating. Late manifestations include diaphoresis, weakness, tremors, anxiety, nausea, and hunger.
- Manifestations resolve after intestine is emptied. However, there is a rapid rise in blood glucose and increase in insulin levels immediately after the intestine empties. This leads to hypoglycemia.

NURSING ACTIONS

- Monitor clients receiving enteral tube feedings and report manifestations of dumping syndrome to the provider.
- Monitor the client for vitamin and mineral deficits (iron and vitamin B_{12}).

CLIENT EDUCATION

- Consume small, frequent meals.
- Consume protein and fat at each meal.
- Avoid food that contains concentrated sugars and restrict lactose intake.
- Plan to consume liquids 1 hr after meals or between meals (no sooner than 30 min after eating).
- Lie down after meals to delay gastric emptying. If reflux is a problem, try a reclining position.

Gastroesophageal reflux disease

- Gastroesophageal reflux disease (GERD) occurs as the result of the abnormal reflux of gastric secretions up the esophagus. This leads to indigestion and heartburn.
- Factors that contribute to GERD include hiatal hernia, obesity, pregnancy, smoking, some medications, and genetics.
- Long-term GERD can cause serious complications, including adenocarcinoma of the esophagus and Barrett's esophagus.
- Manifestations include heartburn, retrosternal burning, painful swallowing, dyspepsia, regurgitation, coughing, hoarseness, and epigastric pain. Pain can be mistaken for a myocardial infarction.

CLIENT EDUCATION

- Avoid situations that lead to increased abdominal pressure, such as wearing tight-fitting clothing.
- Avoid eating for 3 hr before lying down.
- Elevate the body on pillows instead of lying flat and avoid large meals and bedtime snacks.
- Attempt weight loss if overweight or obese.
- Avoid trigger foods (citrus fruits and juices, spicy foods, carbonated beverages).
- Avoid items that reduce lower esophageal sphincter pressure (fatty foods, caffeine, chocolate, alcohol, cigarette smoke, all nicotine products, peppermint and spearmint flavors).

Acute and chronic gastritis

- Gastritis is characterized by inflammation of the gastric mucosa. The gastric mucosa is congested with blood and fluid, becoming inflamed. There is a decrease in acid produced and an overabundance of mucus. Superficial ulcers occur, sometimes leading to hemorrhages.
- Acute gastritis occurs with excessive use of nonsteroidal anti-inflammatory drugs (NSAIDs), bile reflux, ingestion of a strong acid or alkali substance, as a complication of radiation therapy, or as a complication of trauma (burns; food poisoning; severe infection; liver, kidney, or respiratory failure; major surgery).

- Chronic gastritis occurs in the presence of ulcers (benign or malignant), Helicobacter pylori, autoimmune disorders (pernicious anemia), poor diet (excessive caffeine, excessive alcohol intake), medications (alendronate, perindopril), and reflux of pancreatic secretions and bile into stomach.
- Manifestations include abdominal pain or discomfort (can be relieved by eating), headache, lethargy, nausea, anorexia, hiccupping (lasting a few hours to days), heartburn after eating, belching, sour taste in mouth, vomiting, bleeding, and hematemesis (vomiting of blood).
- Acute recovery typically occurs in 1 day but can take 2 to 3 days. The client should eat a bland diet when able to tolerate food. IV fluid replacement therapy is indicated if the condition persists.
- When the condition occurs due to ingestion of strong acids or alkalis, dilution and neutralization of the causal agent is needed. Avoid lavage and emetics due to potential perforation and esophageal damage. Qs

CHRONIC MANAGEMENT: Modify diet, reduce and manage stress, avoid alcohol and NSAIDs. If condition is persistent, the provider will prescribe an H_2 receptor antagonist (famotidine). QEBP

NURSING ACTIONS: Monitor for vitamin deficiency, especially of vitamin B_{12}.

CLIENT EDUCATION

- Avoid eating frequent meals and snacks, as they promote increased gastric acid secretion.
- Avoid alcohol, cigarette smoking, aspirin and other NSAIDs, coffee, black pepper, spicy foods, and caffeine.

Peptic ulcer disease

- Peptic ulcer disease (PUD) is characterized by an erosion of the mucosal layer of the stomach or duodenum. This can be caused by a bacterial infection with *H. pylori* or the chronic use of NSAIDs (aspirin, ibuprofen).
- Some clients who have PUD do not experience manifestations. Others report dull, gnawing pain, burning sensation in the back or low mid-epigastric area, heartburn, constipation or diarrhea, sour taste in mouth, burping, nausea, vomiting, bloating, urea present in breath, and tarry stools. Eating can temporarily relieve pain. Anemia can occur due to blood loss.
- For PUD caused by *H. pylori*, the provider prescribes triple therapy (a combination of antibiotics and acid reducing medications) to be taken for 10 to 14 days.

CLIENT EDUCATION: Avoid coffee, alcohol, caffeine, aspirin and other NSAIDs, cigarette smoking, black pepper, and spicy foods.

Lactose intolerance

- Lactose intolerance results from an inadequate supply of lactase in the intestine, the enzyme that digests lactose.
- The enzyme that converts lactose into glucose, and galactose is absent or insufficient. Manifestations include distention, cramps, flatus, and osmotic diarrhea.
- Small amounts (4 to 6 oz) of milk taken during meals can be tolerated.
- Some dairy products (yogurt, aged cheeses) are low in lactate and can be better tolerated.

NURSING ACTIONS: Monitor for vitamin D and calcium deficiency.

CLIENT EDUCATION
- Avoid or limit intake of foods high in lactose (milk, soft cheese, ice cream, cream soups, sour cream, puddings, coffee creamer).
- Ask the provider about the use of a lactase enzyme.

Ileostomies and colostomies

An ostomy is a surgically created opening on the surface of the abdomen from either the end of the small intestine (ileostomy) or from the colon (colostomy).
- Fluid and electrolyte maintenance is the primary concern for clients who have ileostomies and colostomies.
- The colon absorbs large amounts of fluid, sodium, and potassium.
- Nutrition therapy begins with liquids only and is slowly advanced based upon client tolerance.

NURSING ACTIONS: Provide emotional support to clients due to the risk of altered body image. Qᴘᴄᴄ

CLIENT EDUCATION
- Consume a diet that is high in fluids (at least 1.9 to 2.4 L [64 to 80 oz] per day) and soluble fiber.
- Avoid foods that cause gas (beans, eggs, carbonated beverages), stomal blockage (nuts, raw carrots, popcorn), and foods that produce odor (eggs, fish, garlic).
- Increase intake of calories and protein to promote healing of the stoma site.

Diverticulosis and diverticulitis

Diverticula are pouches protruding through the muscle of the intestinal wall, usually from increased intraluminal pressure. They occur anywhere in the colon, but usually in the sigmoid colon. Unless infection occurs, diverticula cause no problems.
- Diverticulosis is a condition characterized by the presence of diverticula.
- Diverticulitis is inflammation that occurs when fecal matter becomes trapped in the diverticula.
- Manifestations of diverticulitis include abdominal pain, nausea, vomiting, constipation or diarrhea, and fever, accompanied by chills and tachycardia.
- The client receives antibiotics, anticholinergics, and analgesics. Clients who have severe manifestations are admitted to the hospital and dehydration is treated with IV therapy. Opioid analgesics are administered for pain. Complications (peritonitis, bowel obstruction, abscess) can warrant surgical intervention.

- A high-fiber diet can prevent diverticulosis and diverticulitis by producing stools that are easily passed, thus decreasing pressure within the colon.
- During acute diverticulitis, a clear-liquid diet is prescribed until inflammation decreases, then a high-fiber, low-fat diet is indicated.
- Clients require instruction regarding diet adjustment based on the need for an acute intervention or preventive approach.

Inflammatory bowel disease (IBD)

- Crohn's disease (regional enteritis) and ulcerative colitis are chronic, inflammatory bowel diseases characterized by periods of exacerbation and remission.
- Manifestations include nausea, vomiting, abdominal cramps, fever, fatigue, anorexia, weight loss, steatorrhea, and low-grade fever.
- Nutrition therapy is focused on providing nutrients in forms that the client can tolerate.
- A low-residue, high-protein, high-calorie diet with vitamin and mineral supplementation is prescribed during exacerbation to minimize bowel stimulation. Fluid and electrolyte imbalances are corrected with IV fluids or oral replacement fluids.
- Enteral nutrition can be prescribed during exacerbations, especially if the client is reluctant to eat. Because parenteral nutrition is more costly with a relatively similar benefit, it is not used unless enteral nutrition is ineffective or contraindicated.
- When the client is not experiencing an exacerbation, the diet can be broadened based on the client's specific disease process and triggers.

Additional therapy
- Complementary therapies including vitamin C and herbs (flaxseed)
- Yoga, hypnosis, and breathing exercises
- Sedatives
- Antidiarrheal and antiperistaltic agents
- Aminosalicylate medications and corticosteroids to reduce inflammation
- Immunomodulators to alter the immune response and prevent relapse
- Surgery when other treatments are not effective

CLIENT EDUCATION: Avoid intake of substances that cause or exacerbate diarrhea, and avoid nicotine.

Cholecystitis

- Cholecystitis is characterized by inflammation of the gallbladder.
- The gallbladder stores and releases bile that aids in the digestion of fats.
- Manifestations include pain, tenderness, and rigidity in upper right abdomen. Pain can radiate to the right shoulder or midsternal area. Nausea, vomiting, and anorexia also can occur. If the gallbladder becomes filled with pus or becomes gangrenous, perforation can result.
- In clients who have large stones or inability to control the condition with diet modifications, surgery is required.

- Pancreatitis and liver involvement can result from uncontrolled cholecystitis.
- Fat intake should be limited to reduce stimulation of the gallbladder.
- The diet is individualized to the client's needs and tolerance.

Pancreatitis

- Pancreatitis is an inflammation of the pancreas, which can be acute or chronic. In 70% of the acute cases, alcohol use and gallstones are major causes. Chronic pancreatitis can result from acute pancreatitis that does not resolve.
- The pancreas is responsible for secreting enzymes needed to digest fats, carbohydrates, and proteins.
- Nutritional therapy for acute pancreatitis involves reducing pancreatic stimulation. The client is prescribed nothing by mouth (NPO), and a nasogastric tube is inserted to suction gastric contents.
- TPN can be used until oral intake is resumed.
- Nutritional therapy for chronic pancreatitis usually includes a low-fat, high-protein, and high-carbohydrate diet. It can include providing supplements of vitamin C and B-complex vitamins.

Liver disease

- The liver is involved in the metabolism of most nutrients.
- Disorders affecting the liver include cirrhosis, hepatitis, and cancer.
- Malnutrition is common with liver disease.
- Protein needs are increased to promote a positive nitrogen balance and prevent a breakdown of the body's protein stores.
- Carbohydrates are generally not restricted, as they are an important source of calories.
- Caloric requirements might need to be increased based on an evaluation of the client's stage of disease, weight, and general health status.
- Multivitamins (especially vitamins B, C, and K) and mineral supplements might be necessary.
- Alcohol, nicotine, and caffeine should be eliminated.

Celiac disease Qpcc

- Celiac disease is also known as gluten-sensitive enteropathy, celiac sprue, and gluten intolerance.
- It is a chronic, inherited, genetic disorder with autoimmune characteristics. Clients who have celiac disease are unable to digest the protein gluten. They lack the digestive enzyme DPP-IV, which is required to break down the gluten into molecules small enough to be used by the body. In celiac disease, gluten is broken down into peptide strands instead of molecules. The body is not able to metabolize the peptides. If untreated, the client will suffer destruction of the villa and the walls of the small intestine. Celiac disease can go undiagnosed in both children and adults.

- Manifestations vary widely. Children who have celiac disease have diarrhea, steatorrhea, anemia, abdominal distention, impaired growth, lack of appetite, and fatigue. Typical manifestations in adults include diarrhea, abdominal pain, bloating, anemia, steatorrhea, and osteomalacia.
- Treatment for celiac disease is limited to avoiding gluten. However, eliminating gluten, which is found in wheat, rye and barley, is difficult because it is found in many prepared foods. Clients must read food labels carefully in order to adhere to a gluten-free diet. Some gluten-free products are unappealing to clients, and many are more expensive than other products. Prognosis is good for clients who adhere to a gluten-free diet.

NURSING ACTIONS

- Monitor for complications including bleeding (bruising) due to inadequate vitamin K intake, manifestations of anemias (iron, folate, vitamin B_{12}), and manifestations of osteoporosis.
- Collaborate with a dietitian to assist with food selection and label reading.

CLIENT EDUCATION

- Eat foods that are gluten-free (milk, cheese, rice, corn, eggs, potatoes, fruits, vegetables, fresh meats and fish, dried beans).
- Read labels on processed products. Gravy mixes, sauces, cold cuts, soups, and many other products have gluten as an ingredient.
- Read labels and research nonfood products (lipstick, communion wafers, vitamin supplements), which also can have gluten as an ingredient. Qpcc

Active Learning Scenario

A nurse is providing instructions to the guardian of a child who has lactose intolerance. What should the nurse include in the teaching? Use the ATI Active Learning Template: System Disorder to complete this item.

CLIENT EDUCATION

- Describe the underlying cause of lactose intolerance.
- Identify two manifestations of lactose intolerance.
- Identify three foods the child should limit or eliminate from their diet.

Application Exercises

1. A nurse is teaching a client who has constipation about a high-fiber, low-fat diet. Which of the following food choices by the client indicates understanding of the teaching?

   A. Peanut butter

   B. Peeled apples

   C. Hardboiled egg

   D. Brown rice

2. A nurse is assessing a client who is postoperative from a gastric bypass and who just finished eating a meal. Which of the following findings are manifestations of dumping syndrome? (Select all that apply.)

   A. Bradycardia

   B. Dizziness

   C. Dry skin

   D. Hypotension

   E. Diarrhea

3. A nurse is collecting data from a client who has peptic ulcer disease (PUD). Which of the following findings should the nurse expect? (Select all that apply.)

   A. Steatorrhea

   B. Anemia

   C. Tarry stools

   D. Epigastric pain

   E. Swollen lymph nodes

4. A nurse is reviewing information about following a low-fat diet, with a client who is recovering from pancreatitis. Which of the following foods should the nurse recommend? (Select all that apply.)

   A. Ribeye steak

   B. Oatmeal

   C. Ice cream

   D. Canned peaches

   E. Pretzels

5. A nurse is instructing a client who has celiac disease about foods to avoid. Which of the following foods should the nurse include in the teaching?

   A. Potatoes

   B. Graham crackers

   C. Wild rice

   D. Canned pears

Application Exercises Key

1. D. **CORRECT:** When evaluating outcomes, the nurse should recognize that the client indicates understanding about a high-fiber, low-fat diet by choosing brown rice as food that is a good source of fiber and is low in fat.

   Ⓝ *NCLEX® Connection: Basic Care and Comfort, Elimination*

2. B, D, E. **CORRECT:** The nurse should analyze cues when monitoring the client who is postoperative following gastric bypass and just finished eating a meal and determine that when a portion of the stomach is no longer available to serve as a reservoir, a large amount of food is rapidly dumped into the small intestine, and fluid shifts from general circulation into the intestine. This can result in the manifestations of dizziness and hypotension due to a decrease in circulating volume, and diarrhea can occur from increased peristalsis.

   Ⓝ *NCLEX® Connection: Basic Care and Comfort, Elimination*

3. B, C, D. **CORRECT:** The nurse should recognize cues from the client's data collection and identify that iron deficiency anemia due to blood loss, tarry stools due to intestinal bleeding, and epigastric pain described as a gnawing or burning sensation can be clinical findings of PUD.

   Ⓝ *NCLEX® Connection: Basic Care and Comfort, Elimination*

4. B, D, E. **CORRECT:** When taking actions and reviewing low-fat diet information with a client who is recovering from pancreatitis, the nurse should include that oatmeal, canned peaches, and pretzels are sources of easily digested carbohydrates that are low in fat.

   Ⓝ *NCLEX® Connection: Basic Care and Comfort, Nutrition and Oral Hydration*

5. B. **CORRECT:** When taking actions and instructing a client who has celiac disease about foods to avoid, the nurse should include that graham crackers are made from wheat flour and a client who has celiac disease should avoid products that are made from wheat flour.

   Ⓝ *NCLEX® Connection: Basic Care and Comfort, Nutrition and Oral Hydration*

Active Learning Scenario Key

Using the ATI Active Learning Template: System Disorder

CLIENT EDUCATION

- The underlying cause of lactose intolerance is an inadequate level of lactase. The enzyme that converts lactose into glucose and galactose is absent or insufficient.
- Manifestations
  - Abdominal distension
  - Cramps
  - Flatus
  - Diarrhea
- Foods to limit or avoid include milk, soft cheese, ice cream, cream soups, puddings.

Ⓝ *NCLEX® Connection: Physiological Adaptation, Illness Management*

UNIT 3   ALTERATIONS IN NUTRITION

CHAPTER 15 *Renal Disorders*

Nurses should understand the nutritional needs of clients who have renal disorders. It is important to explore dietary needs with the client and recommend modifications related to the disease process. Understanding the role of primary and secondary prevention is essential to successful treatment.

The kidneys have two primary functions: maintaining blood volume and excreting waste products. Other functions include the regulation of acid-base balance, blood pressure, calcium and phosphorous metabolism, and red blood cell production. Kidney damage and/or loss of kidney function have profound effects on the client's nutritional state. Urea is a waste by-product of protein metabolism, and urea levels rise with kidney disease. Monitoring protein intake is critical.

Short-term kidney disease requires nutritional support for healing rather than dietary restrictions. Dietary recommendations are dependent upon the stage of kidney disease.

Nutritional considerations included in this chapter are for chronic kidney disease and end-stage kidney disease, acute kidney injury, nephrotic syndrome, and nephrolithiasis (kidney stones).

Referral to and consultation with a registered dietitian to determine calories, protein, and other nutrients is essential for the client to decrease the risk of malnutrition.

ASSESSMENT/DATA COLLECTION

Chronic kidney disease is distinguished by an increase in blood creatinine. Manifestations include fatigue, back pain, and appetite changes. It is a progressive disorder, characterized by five stages.
- Stage 1: at risk for CKD
- Stage 2: mild CKD
- Stage 3: moderate CKD
- Stage 4: severe CKD
- Stage 5: CKD requiring dialysis or transplant for survival (end-stage kidney disease)

End-stage kidney disease (ESKD) manifestations include fatigue, decreased alertness, anemia, decreased urination, headache, and weight loss.

Acute kidney injury (AKI) manifestations include a decrease in urination, decreased sensation in the extremities, swelling of the lower extremities, and flank pain. It is characterized by rising blood levels of urea and other nitrogenous wastes.

Nephrotic syndrome's most pronounced manifestations are edema and high proteinuria. Other manifestations include hypoalbuminemia, hyperlipidemia, and blood hypercoagulation.

Kidney stones are characterized by sudden, intense pain that is typically located in the flank and is unrelieved by position changes as the stone moves out of the kidney pelvis and down the ureter. Diaphoresis, nausea, and vomiting are common, and there can be blood in the urine. The majority of kidney stones are made of calcium oxalate.

NUTRITIONAL GUIDELINES AND NURSING INTERVENTIONS

General renal considerations

- Monitor kidney parameters for clients who have renal disorders.
  - Nurses should monitor weight daily or as prescribed. Weight is an indicator of fluid status, which is a primary concern. ○EBP
  - Monitor fluid intake and encourage compliance with fluid restrictions.
  - Nurses should monitor urine output. Placement of an indwelling urinary catheter might be necessary for accurate measurement.
  - Monitor for manifestations of constipation. Fluid restrictions predispose clients to constipation.
- Explain why dietary changes are necessary. Alterations in the intake of protein, calories, sodium, potassium, phosphorus, and other vitamins are required.
- Provide support for the client and family.

Chronic kidney disease (stages 1 to 4)

- Stages 1 to 4 are predialysis and characterized by increasing blood creatinine levels and a decreasing glomerular filtration rate (GFR).

THERAPEUTIC NUTRITION

- Goals of nutritional therapy
  - Slow the progression of CKD.
  - Control blood glucose and hypertension.
  - Help preserve remaining kidney function by limiting the intake of protein, which results in decreased phosphorus levels.
- Restricting phosphorus intake slows the progression of kidney disease. High levels of phosphorus contribute to calcium and phosphorus deposits in the kidneys.
- Protein restriction is essential for clients who have stages 1 to 4 CKD.
  - Slows the progression of kidney disease.
  - Too little protein results in the breakdown of body protein. Carefully determine protein intake.

DIETARY RECOMMENDATIONS

- Restrict sodium intake to maintain blood pressure.
- Restrict potassium intake to prevent hyperkalemia.
- The recommended daily protein intake is 0.8 to 1.0 g/kg/day of ideal body weight.
  - Protein restrictions are decreased as the disease progresses to ESKD, and to decrease the workload on the kidneys.
  - High biologic value proteins are recommended for clients who have CKD to prevent catabolism of muscle tissue. These proteins include eggs, meats, poultry, game, fish, soy, and dairy products.
- Limit meat intake to 5 to 6 oz/day for most males and 4 oz/day for most females.
- Limit dairy products to 1/2; cup per day.
- Limit high-phosphorus foods (peanut butter, dried peas and beans, bran, cola, chocolate, beer, some whole grains) to one serving or less per day.
- Caution clients to use vitamin and mineral supplements only when recommended by a provider. Avoid high protein sports drinks, energy drinks, or meal supplements. Avoid herbal supplements that can affect bleeding time and blood pressure. Qs

End-stage kidney disease

ESKD, or stage 5 CKD, occurs when the GFR is less than 15 mL/min and the blood creatinine level steadily rises, indicating complete kidney failure.

THERAPEUTIC NUTRITION

- The goal of nutritional therapy is to maintain appropriate fluid status, blood pressure, and blood chemistries.
  - A low-protein, low-phosphorus, low-potassium, low-sodium (2 to 3 g/day), fluid-restricted diet is recommended.
  - Consume adequate calories (35 kcal/kg of body weight) to maintain body protein stores.

- Monitor potassium level and replace as needed. Sodium and fluid allowances are determined by blood pressure, weight, blood electrolyte findings, and urine output.
- Achieving a well-balanced diet based on the above guidelines is difficult. The National Renal Diet provides clients with a list of food choices.
- Protein needs increase from 0.6 to 1.0 g/kg prior to dialysis to 1.0 to 1.2 g/kg/day or higher once dialysis has begun because protein and amino acids are lost in the dialysate, depending on the type of dialysis.
  - Fifty percent of protein intake should come from biologic sources (eggs, milk, meat, fish, poultry, soy).
- Restrict phosphorus (700 to 1,200 mg/day).
  - A high protein requirement leads to an increase in phosphorus intake.
  - Foods high in phosphorus are milk products, beef liver, chocolate, nuts, and legumes.
  - Phosphate binders (calcium carbonate, calcium acetate) are taken with all meals and snacks.
- Vitamin D deficiency occurs as the kidneys are unable to convert vitamin D to its active form.
  - This alters the metabolism of calcium, phosphorus, and magnesium, leading to hyperphosphatemia, hypocalcemia, and hypermagnesemia.
  - Calcium supplements will likely be required because foods high in phosphorus (which are restricted) are also high in calcium.

Acute kidney injury

AKI is an abrupt, rapid decline in kidney function caused by trauma, sepsis, poor perfusion, or medications, and usually is reversible. AKI can cause hyponatremia, hyperkalemia, hypocalcemia, and hyperphosphatemia. Fluid overload leading to pulmonary edema is a complication of AKI.

THERAPEUTIC NUTRITION

- Diet therapy for AKI is dependent upon the phase of AKI and its underlying cause. Protein, calories, fluids, potassium, and sodium need to be individualized according to the three phases of AKI (oliguric, diuretic, recovery) and whether the client is receiving dialysis.
- Recommendation is to consume 20 to 30 cal/kg/day of body weight in clients who are in any stage of AKI to maintain energy and demands of stress.
- Simple carbohydrates, fats, oils, and low-protein starches are included in the diet. Provide nonprotein calories in an adequate amount to maintain the client's weight.
- Protein intake can increase to 1.0 to 1.2 g/kg/day or higher if the client is receiving dialysis, compared to 0.6 g/kg (40 g/day) for nondialysis clients.
- Potassium and sodium are dependent on urine output, blood values, and if the client is receiving dialysis.
  - Potassium is restricted to 60 to 70 mEq/day when on dialysis.
  - Sodium is restricted to 1 to 2 g/day if not receiving dialysis, and 2 to 4 g/day if receiving dialysis, which also depends on the phase.
  - Calcium requirements are less than 2,000 mg daily if receiving hemodialysis or peritoneal dialysis.
- Fluids are restricted to the client's daily urine output plus 500 mL during the oliguric phase. Fluid needs are increased during the diuretic phase.

Nephrotic syndrome

- Nephrotic syndrome results in the increased excretion of proteins into the urine, resulting in hypoalbuminemia, edema, hyperlipidemia, and blood hypercoagulation. Prolonged protein loss leads to protein malnutrition, anemia, and vitamin D deficiency.
- Diabetes mellitus, kidney damage due to medications or chemicals, autoimmune disorders, and infections can cause nephrotic syndrome.

THERAPEUTIC NUTRITION

- Nutritional therapy goals include minimizing edema, replacing lost nutrients, minimizing kidney damage, controlling hypertension, and preventing protein malnutrition that can lead to muscle catabolism.
- Dietary recommendations indicate sufficient protein and low sodium intake.
  - Adequate amount of protein intake is 0.7 to 1.0 g/kg/day.
  - Soy-based proteins can decrease protein losses and lower blood lipid levels.
  - Low-sodium diet of 2,000 mg/day can help control edema and hypertension.
  - Carbohydrates should provide the majority of the client's daily calories.
  - Cholesterol, trans fats, and saturated fats can be restricted to assist in controlling high lipid levels.
  - Provide a multiple vitamin supplement to replace loss of vitamins with protein excretion. Replace loss of vitamin D with a supplement as needed.

Nephrolithiasis

- The most common type of kidney stone is made of calcium oxalate.
- Contributing factors include inadequate fluid intake, elevated urine pH, and excess excretion through the kidneys of oxalate, calcium, and uric acid.
- Kidney stone formation is more influenced by the amount of oxalate in the client's system than calcium. A client who has an ileostomy has an increased risk of kidney stones.

Preventative nutrition: Excessive intake of protein, sodium, calcium, and oxalates (rhubarb, spinach, beets) can increase the risk of stone formation.

THERAPEUTIC NUTRITION

- Increasing fluid consumption is the primary intervention for the treatment and prevention of kidney stones. Daily fluid intake should be enough to produce at least 2 L of urine per day. Drink some fluid before bedtime because urine becomes more concentrated at night. This is particularly important for clients who have cystine stones, which requires an even greater daily fluid intake.
- Recommendation for calcium oxalate stone formation is to limit animal protein, excess sodium, alcohol, and caffeine use. Low potassium can contribute to calcium stone formation.
- Foods high in oxalates include spinach, rhubarb, beets, nuts, chocolate, tea, wheat bran, and strawberries, and should be limited in the diet. Avoid megadoses of vitamin C, which increase the amount of oxalate excreted.
- Recommendation for prevention of uric acid stones is to limit foods high in purines, which include lean meats, organ meats, whole grains, and legumes.

Application Exercises

1. A nurse is teaching a client who has stage 2 chronic kidney disease about dietary management. Which of the following information should the nurse include in the instructions?

    A. Restrict protein intake.

    B. Maintain a high-phosphorus diet.

    C. Increase intake of foods high in potassium.

    D. Limit dairy products to 1 cup/day.

2. A nurse is planning care for a client who has ESKD. Which of the following should the nurse include in the plan of care? (Select all that apply.)

    A. Monitor the client's weight daily.

    B. Encourage the client to comply with fluid restrictions.

    C. Evaluate intake and output.

    D. Instruct the client on restricting calories from carbohydrates.

    E. Monitor for constipation.

3. A nurse is teaching a client about protein needs when on dialysis. Which of the following instructions should the nurse include in the teaching? (Select all that apply.)

    A. Consume 1.0 to 1.2 g/kg/day to maintain body protein stores.

    B. Take phosphate binders when eating protein-rich foods.

    C. Calcium intake should be less than 800 mg/day.

    D. Drink fluids that are at a room temperature.

    E. Consume the majority of daily protein intake in the morning.

4. A nurse is teaching about diet restrictions to a client who has acute kidney injury and is on hemodialysis. Which of the following recommendations should the nurse include in the teaching?

    A. Calorie intake of 20 to 30 cal/kg

    B. Decrease total fat intake to 45% of daily calories.

    C. Decrease potassium intake to 100 to 130 mEq/kg.

    D. Limit sodium intake to 4.5 g/day.

5. A nurse is completing discharge teaching about diet and fluid restrictions to a client who has a calcium oxalate-based kidney stone. Which of the following instructions should the nurse include in the teaching?

    A. Drink at least 2L/day..

    B. Decrease calcium intake to less than 400 mg/day.

    C. Increase intake of vitamin C supplements.

    D. Limit consumption of purine substances.

Application Exercises Key

1. A. **CORRECT:** When taking actions and teaching a client who has stage 2 CKD about dietary management, the nurse should instruct the client that restricting protein intake decreases the risk for proteinuria and decreases the workload on the kidney.

   Ⓝ *NCLEX® Connection: Basic Care and Comfort, Nutrition and Oral Hydration*

2. A, B, C, E. **CORRECT:** When a nurse is taking actions and planning care for a client who has ESKD, the nurse should include the interventions of monitoring the client's daily weight which assists in determining fluid retention and encouraging the client to comply with fluid restrictions which can help slow fluid retention. The nurse should include evaluating I&O to assist with determining if there is an increase in fluid retention and monitoring the client for constipation which can occur because of fluid restrictions..

   Ⓝ *NCLEX® Connection: Basic Care and Comfort, Nutrition and Oral Hydration*

3. A, B, C. **CORRECT:** When a nurse is taking actions and teaching a client about protein needs when on dialysis, the nurse should instruct the client to maintain protein stores, the client should consume 1.0 to 1.2 g/kg/day. The nurse should also include that protein consumption increases phosphorus intake and that phosphate binders are recommended with meals. The nurse should teach the client that calcium intake should be less than 800 mg/day.

   Ⓝ *NCLEX® Connection: Basic Care and Comfort, Nutrition and Oral Hydration*

4. A. **CORRECT:** When taking actions and teaching the client who has acute kidney injury and is on hemodialysis about dietary restrictions, the nurse should instruct the client to maintain a calorie intake of 20 to 30 cal/kg.

   Ⓝ *NCLEX® Connection: Basic Care and Comfort, Nutrition and Oral Hydration*

5. A. **CORRECT:** When taking actions and providing discharge teaching about diet and fluid restrictions to a client who has a calcium oxalate-based kidney stone, the nurse should teach the client to drink at least 2 L/day

   Ⓝ *NCLEX® Connection: Health Promotion and Maintenance, Health Promotion/Disease Prevention*

Active Learning Scenario

A nurse is reviewing teaching for a client who has nephrotic syndrome. What information should the nurse include? Use the ATI Active Learning Template: System Disorder to complete this item.

ALTERATION IN HEALTH (DIAGNOSIS)

COMPLICATIONS: List three.

CLIENT EDUCATION: Include five teaching points.

Active Learning Scenario Key

Using the ATI Active Learning Template: System Disorder

ALTERATION IN HEALTH (DIAGNOSIS): Nephrotic syndrome is a renal disorder in which there is increased excretion of proteins into the urine.

COMPLICATIONS
- Hypoalbuminemia
- Proteinuria
- Edema
- Hyperlipidemia
- Malnutrition
- Anemia

CLIENT EDUCATION
- Increase protein intake to prevent catabolism of muscle tissue.
- Limit sodium intake to control edema and hypertension.
- Consume foods low in trans fats and cholesterol.
- Consume foods high in carbohydrates to increase calorie intake.
- Take a vitamin supplement to replace vitamin loss that occurs with protein excretion.

Ⓝ *NCLEX® Connection: Physiological Adaptation, Illness Management*

UNIT 3   ALTERATIONS IN NUTRITION

CHAPTER 16 *Diabetes Mellitus*

Glucose is the body's primary source of energy, and insulin is needed to assist the body in the breakdown of glucose to a form that is used for energy. Diabetes mellitus inhibits the body's production and/or use of insulin. This results in elevated blood glucose levels. Complications of diabetes mellitus are characterized as macrovascular (cardiovascular and cerebrovascular disease) or microvascular (kidney, nerve, and vision problems). For clients who are pregnant, blood glucose control prevents maternal and fetal complications.

The nurse assists the client in identifying lifestyle changes necessary to manage diabetes mellitus, including diet and activity level.

TYPES OF DIABETES MELLITUS

Prediabetes

- Clients who have glucose levels that are elevated above the expected range but below the diagnostic criteria for diabetes mellitus are said to have prediabetes.
- Clients who have prediabetes are encouraged to adopt lifestyle modifications to prevent the development of diabetes mellitus.

Type 1 diabetes mellitus

- Autoimmune disease is triggered by genetic links or a viral infection.
- Damage to or destruction of beta cells of the pancreas results in an absence of insulin production.
- Most often diagnosed before 18 years of age; can occur at any age

Type 2 diabetes mellitus

- Results from genetic and environmental factors
- Characterized by altered patterns of insulin secretion and decreased cellular uptake of glucose (insulin resistance)

Gestational diabetes mellitus (GDM)

- Glucose intolerance that is recognized during pregnancy and typically resolves after birth.
- Clients who have a history of GDM have an increased risk for developing diabetes mellitus type 2 later in life.

ASSESSMENT/DATA COLLECTION

Hypoglycemia is a blood glucose level less than 70 mg/dL. It results from too much insulin intake, inadequate food intake, delayed or skipped meals, extra physical activity, or consumption of alcohol without food. Manifestations include mild shakiness, mental confusion, sweating, palpitations, headache, lack of coordination, blurred vision, seizures, and coma.

Hyperglycemia is a blood glucose level above the expected reference range. It results from an imbalance with food, medication, and activity, combined with an inadequate amount of insulin production or cells that are insulin-resistant.

- Infection, other illness, and stress can cause an increase in blood glucose.
- Primary manifestations include polydipsia (excessive thirst), polyuria (excessive urination), and polyphagia (excess hunger and eating). As hyperglycemia progresses, ketones (which can be detected in the urine) and other manifestations (hyperventilation [Kussmaul respirations], dehydration, fruity odor to the breath, headache, inability to concentrate, decreased levels of consciousness, seizures leading to coma) develop.
- The Somogyi phenomenon is morning hyperglycemia in response to overnight hypoglycemia. Providing a bedtime snack and appropriate insulin dose prevents this phenomenon.
- The dawn phenomenon is an elevation of blood glucose around 0500 to 0600. It results from an overnight release of growth hormone and is treated by increasing the amount of insulin provided during the overnight hours.

Metabolic syndrome is a cluster of factors that increase the risk for diabetes mellitus and cardiovascular complications. Factors include elevated glucose levels, central obesity, hyperlipidemia, hypertension, and low levels of HDL cholesterol. The presence of at least 3 factors indicates metabolic syndrome.

NUTRITIONAL GUIDELINES AND NURSING INTERVENTIONS

Hypoglycemia

- Clients who have hypoglycemia should take 15 g of a readily absorbable carbohydrate. Qs
  - Four glucose tablets (5 g each)
  - Five to six hard candies
  - ½ cup (4 oz) juice or regular soda
  - 1 tbsp honey or sugar
- Retest the blood glucose in 15 min. If it is less than 70 mg/dL, repeat the above steps. Once levels stabilize, have the client take an additional carbohydrate and protein snack or small meal, depending on the severity of the hypoglycemic episode and whether the next meal is more than 1 hr away.

Hyperglycemia

Clients who have hyperglycemia should do the following.
- Notify the provider or go to the emergency department for difficulty concentrating, altered consciousness, or seizure activity.
- Take medication if forgotten.

GENERAL NUTRITIONAL GUIDELINES

- Coronary heart disease (CHD) is a frequent cause of death among clients who have diabetes. Clients who have diabetes are encouraged to follow a diet that is high in fiber and low in saturated fat, trans fat, and cholesterol to prevent CHD.
- Dietary intake should be individualized according to the client's individual needs, need for weight management, and lipid and glucose patterns. Clients should space food intake throughout the day (regular meals and a snack or snacks). General guidelines follow.
  - **Carbohydrates**
    - Teach carbohydrate counting to the client and assist the client with their individual meal plan based on their calorie needs which specifies the number of carbohydrate choices to eat with each meal and or snack.
    - Encourage the client to consume carbohydrates found in grains, fruits, legumes, and milk. Limit simple carbohydrates, which include refined grains and sugars.
  - **Fats**
    - Clients should eat less saturated and trans fats.
    - Polyunsaturated fatty acids are found in fish. Two or more servings per week are recommended.
    - Consuming foods enriched with plant sterols or stanols can reduce LDL cholesterol.
  - **Fiber**
    - Promote fiber intake (beans, vegetables, oats, whole grains) to improve carbohydrate metabolism and lower cholesterol.
    - Recommendation for fiber intake includes at least 14 g per 1,000 calories.
  - **Protein:** Protein from meats, eggs, fish, nuts, beans, and soy products should comprise 15% to 20% of total caloric intake. Reduce protein intake if needed in clients who have diabetes and kidney failure.
  - **Sodium:** Limit to 2,300 mg/day.
- Encourage clients to eliminate all tobacco use due to the increased risk of cardiovascular disease.
- Moderate alcohol intake can lower the risk for cardiovascular disease. Clients should limit daily alcohol intake to one alcoholic beverage for females or two for males.
  - To avoid hypoglycemia, the client should consume alcohol with a meal or immediately after a meal.
  - Alcoholic beverages should not replace food intake.
- Vitamin and mineral requirements are unchanged for clients who have diabetes. Supplements are recommended for identified deficiencies.

- Artificial sweeteners are acceptable (sucralose, aspartame, saccharin, acesulfame, potassium). Sugar alcohols (xylitol, mannitol, sorbitol) contain some sugar, but not as much as natural sweeteners. Sucrose (table sugar) can be included in a diabetic diet and should be counted in the total calories for the day to ensure antidiabetic medications are sufficient to cover intake.
- Cultural and personal preferences should be considered in planning food intake. Qpcc
- According to the American Diabetes Association and the Academy of Dietetics and Nutrition, daily nutritional requirements are based on the needs of each client.
- A dietitian works with the client to develop meal planning that meets the client's needs based on healthy food choices. The goal of therapy is to maintain blood glucose levels as close to the expected reference range as possible. Qtc
  - The dietitian instructs the client on various dietary methods, including exchange list and carbohydrate counting.
- Using the Food Lists for Diabetes (formerly called Exchange Lists) as a guide for meal planning allows for the incorporation of three basic food groups: protein, carbohydrates, and fats.
  - Each client has a recommended number of daily exchanges within each group based on the client's needs.

Carbohydrate counting

Carbohydrate counting focuses on counting total grams of carbohydrates in each food item. Many clients find it easier than exchange lists because of the simplicity and flexibility. It does not require the client to learn how much a portion size is.
- One serving equals 15 g of carbohydrates. Clients are free to choose what carbohydrates to consume but are encouraged to choose a variety of types and include consistent amounts of protein and fats in the diet.
  - Foods that contain 15 g of carbohydrates
    - 1 slice of sandwich bread
    - 1/2 cup cooked pasta
    - 1/2 cup canned fruit in juice (not syrup)
    - 1/4 cup dried fruit
    - 3 cups raw vegetables
    - 1 1/2 cup cooked vegetables
    - 4 to 6 snack crackers
    - 1/2 cup regular ice cream
- With basic carbohydrate counting, a client consumes a specific amount or servings of carbohydrates at each meal and snack.
- With advanced carbohydrate counting, clients calculate mealtime insulin based on the amount of carbohydrates consumed. Clients must be able to perform basic math skills and be willing to check their glucose before each meal to provide a corrective insulin dose if the glucose level is too high.
- Clients can exchange carbohydrate selections as long as the grams of carbohydrates are the same per serving. Food selections can vary in the amount of additional calories from fat and protein each food can contain.

OTHER NURSING INTERVENTIONS

- Provide instructions to the client on the following, and discuss these at subsequent appointments. Q EBP
  - Self-monitoring of blood glucose
  - Dietary and activity recommendations
  - Manifestations and treatment of hypoglycemia and hyperglycemia, to include the importance of taking medications as prescribed
  - Long-term complications of diabetes
  - Psychological implications
  - Community organizations and support groups whose focus is diabetes

- Children who have diabetes require guardian/caregiver support, guidance, and participation. Dietary intake must provide for proper growth and development. Altered nutritional needs during times of growth and fluctuations in eating patterns and activity levels can make management complicated. Q PCC
- For older adult clients, ask questions to determine the presence of deficits that impede adequate nutrition or safe medication administration (cognitive impairment, vision and hearing changes, altered dentition, anorexia, financial barriers).
- For pregnant clients, there must be a balance between maternal blood glucose goals and nutritional needs of pregnancy. Clients might have to monitor blood glucose more often (up to eight times daily).
- Teach proper calibration and use of the self-monitoring of blood glucose, record keeping, and reporting of levels to health care provider.

16.1 Case study

Scenario introduction

A client who has a recent diagnosis of type 2 diabetes mellitus is at the provider's office for an education session with the nurse.

Scene 1

Client: There is so much information to learn; I am glad we have this time to talk.

Nurse: I am here to answer your questions. Did you bring a list with you?

Client: I did, and a pencil to take notes.

Nurse: Excellent! Let's get started.

Scene 2

The client reviews their list of questions with the nurse.

Client: I would like to review some information about artificial sweeteners.

Nurse: It is best to use nonnutritive sweeteners such as saccharin, aspartame and sucralose and try to drink water instead of sugar-sweetened and nonnutritive-sweetened beverages.

Client: That is very helpful, I can look for that information on the food label.

Scene 3

The client continues to review their list of questions with the nurse.

Client: I really like to drink beer when I am out with the guys. Will that be a problem if I switch to light beer?

Nurse: If you decide to drink beer, you can reduce your risk of a low blood sugar that night if you eat food while drinking. It's important to remember that moderate alcohol intake can still have long term detrimental effects on blood glucose control.

Client: Guess I was expecting that, since we discussed my meal plan in such detail.

Nurse: Yes, I'm glad you have a better understanding now of what a serving of carbohydrates really looks like.

Scenario conclusion

The client leaves the office with a list of notes and thanks the nurse for answering their questions.

Case study exercises

1. The nurse is evaluating their discussion regarding nonnutritive sweeteners. The nurse identifies the client understands the teaching when they select which of the following choices of sweeteners to use? Select all that apply.

   A. Sucrose
   B. Aspartame
   C. Mannitol
   D. Xylitol
   E. Sucralose

2. The nurse is reinforcing dietary teaching with the client. Which of the following information should the nurse include?

   A. Carbohydrates counting is vital to the meal planning approach.
   B. Use hydrogenated oils for cooking.
   C. Choose whole grains for choices of fiber.
   D. Eat something if choosing to drink alcohol.
   E. Never estimate portion sizes, always have an exact measuring tool.

3. The nurse is reviewing the teaching session with the client. Which of the following client statements indicates understanding?

   A. "I will avoid having snacks."
   B. "I can't eat anything containing sugar."
   C. "I will eat a variety of different foods to get my daily carbohydrates."
   D. "I will not eat more than 2,800 mg of sodium a day."

CLIENT EDUCATION

- Exercise as appropriate and when blood glucose levels are within an acceptable range. Closely monitor blood glucose; decreased medication doses might be required with strenuous exercise to prevent hypoglycemia.
  - Recommendations for adults who have diabetes mellitus includes exercising at least 3 days/week for 150 min total.
  - Adults should not sit for more than 90 min at a time.
- Lose weight if appropriate. It is important for clients who have type 2 diabetes mellitus and have a BMI greater than 25, as it can decrease insulin resistance, improve glucose and lipid levels, and lower blood pressure.
  - Successful weight loss programs include managing calorie intake, exercising, and making lifestyle modifications.
- Be aware of the timing for antidiabetic medications in regard to food intake (before or with meals, or regardless of calorie intake). Take medications at the appropriate time for maximum therapeutic effect.
- Perform self-monitoring of blood glucose. Strict control of glucose can reduce or postpone complications (retinopathy, nephropathy, neuropathy).
- Obtain regular evaluations from the provider.

Active Learning Scenario

A nurse is reviewing the discharge plan for a client who has type 1 diabetes mellitus. How should the nurse use interprofessional care in the plan? Use the ATI Active Learning Template: System Disorder to complete this item.

INTERPROFESSIONAL CARE: Describe the role of the registered dietitian on the health care team.

CLIENT EDUCATION: Describe three teaching points offered by this member of the registered dietitian.

Active Learning Scenario Key

Using the ATI Active Learning Template: System Disorder

INTERPROFESSIONAL CARE: Registered dietitian: Development of meal planning based on healthy food choices to meet the client's needs.

CLIENT EDUCATION

- Review of the food lists for diabetes: Incorporate proteins, carbohydrates, and fats within each group based on the client's needs.
- Review of carbohydrate counting: Consider the total grams of carbohydrates in each food item and the quantity needed for each meal and snack.
- Review information on food labels: Teach how to read food labels to identify amounts of carbohydrates contained in food.

Ⓝ *NCLEX® Connection: Physiological Adaptation, Illness Management*

Application Exercises

1. A nurse is assessing a client who is has hypoglycemia. Which of the following findings should the nurse expect?
   - A. Fruity breath odor
   - B. Diaphoresis
   - C. Ketones in urine
   - D. Polyuria

2. A nurse is caring for a client who has diabetes mellitus and reports feeling shaky and weak. The client's blood glucose is 53 mg/dL. Which of the following actions should the nurse take?
   - A. Provide subcutaneous insulin for the client.
   - B. Offer the client 120 mL (4 oz) fruit juice.
   - C. Give the client IV potassium.
   - D. Administer IV sodium bicarbonate.

Application Exercises Key

1. C. **CORRECT:** The nurse should recognize cues from the client's history and expect that a client who is experiencing hypoglycemia can have diaphoresis and cool, clammy skin.

   Ⓝ *NCLEX® Connection: Reduction of Risk Potential, System-Specific Assessments*

2. B. **CORRECT:** When taking actions to treat a client who has manifestations of hypoglycemia, the nurse should offer the client 15 g of carbohydrate, such as 120 mL fruit juice.

   Ⓝ *NCLEX® Connection: Reduction of Risk Potential, System-Specific Assessments*

Case Study Exercises Key

1. B, E. **CORRECT:** When evaluating client teaching, the nurse should identify that the client understands the use of nonnutritive sweeteners by selecting aspartame and sucralose as acceptable artificial sweeteners that can sweeten foods and beverages without adding calories.

   Ⓝ *NCLEX® Connection: Physiological Adaptation, Illness Management*

2. A, C, E. **CORRECT:** When taking actions and reinforcing dietary teaching with this client, the nurse should remind the client of the importance of carbohydrate counting when meal planning, to choose whole grains for fiber options and since the client admitted to drinking beer, the nurse should reinforce with the client to eat food if consuming alcohol.

   Ⓝ *NCLEX® Connection: Physiological Adaptation, Illness Management*

3. C. **CORRECT:** To avoid extra carbohydrate intake, the client should eat fruit that was canned with water or juice rather than syrup, honey, or molasses.

   Ⓝ *NCLEX® Connection: Basic Care and Comfort, Nutrition and Oral Hydration*

UNIT 3   ALTERATIONS IN NUTRITION

CHAPTER 17 # Cancer and Immunosuppression Disorders

Nurses should be knowledgeable of nutritional needs for clients who have cancer and immunosuppression disorders. Cancer and cancer treatments can affect chewing, swallowing, satiety, digestion, taste, appetite, nutrient absorption, use of glucose, and stool formation (dependent on type).

Protein-calorie malnutrition and body wasting are common secondary diagnoses for clients who have cancer or immunosuppression disorders (HIV/AIDS). Nutritional deficits are a major cause of morbidity and mortality for these clients. Adverse effects of treatments compromise the nutritional status of affected clients. Immunosuppression disorders increase the body's metabolic demands. Alterations in fat storage and metabolism are related to medications used in treatment of the disorder. While subcutaneous fat is lost in the face and extremities, fatty deposits occur in the liver and skeletal muscles, which is called lipodystrophy.

The goals of nutritional therapy are to minimize the nutritional complications of disease, improve nutritional status, prevent muscle wasting, maintain weight, promote healing, reduce adverse effects, decrease morbidity and mortality, and enhance quality of life and overall effectiveness of treatment therapies. Nutritional plans are individualized for client needs.

ASSESSMENT/DATA COLLECTION

- Current illness and presence of other medical diagnoses
- Nutritional habits, food preferences, and restrictions
- Food allergies
- Height, weight, body mass index (BMI), weight trends

RISK FACTORS

Immunosuppression disorders

- Unprotected sex (HIV)
- Use of contaminated needles (injection substance use [HIV])
- Use of medications that have immunosuppressive effects (cytotoxic medications, corticosteroids, disease modifying immunosuppressive medications)
- History of radiation treatment
- Congenital immune deficiencies

Cancer

- Obesity
- Excessive fat intake
- Sedentary lifestyle
- Consumption of processed meats, red meats, refined grains
- Excessive alcohol intake
- Family history
- History of cigarette smoking

LABORATORY TESTS

Prealbumin, albumin, ferritin, transferrin

NUTRITIONAL GUIDELINES AND NURSING INTERVENTIONS

Immunosuppression

- Monitor the effectiveness of nutrition (weight, BMI, laboratory findings).
- Assist the client to set realistic goals for nutrition and food consumption.
- Instruct the client on strategies to manage adverse effects of treatment.

CLIENT EDUCATION: Make food choices based on nutrition recommendations.

Cancer

Excess body fat stimulates the production of estrogen and progesterone, which can intensify the growth of various cell types and can contribute to breast, gallbladder, colon, prostate, uterine, and kidney cancers.

NURSING ACTIONS: Use semisolid, thickened foods for clients who have dysphagia, and instruct them to sit upright and tilt their head forward when swallowing. Qs

CLIENT EDUCATION

- Eat more on days when feeling better (on "good" days).
- Consume nutritional supplements that are high in protein and/or calories as between-meal snacks. When necessary, use as a meal replacement.
- Increase protein and caloric content of foods.
  - Substitute whole milk for water in recipes.
  - Add milk, cheese, yogurt, or ice cream to dishes.
  - Use peanut butter as a spread for fruits.
  - Use yogurt as a topping for fruit.
  - Dip meats in eggs, milk, and breadcrumbs before cooking.
- **Preventative nutrition**
  - Consume adequate dietary fiber (25 to 38 g/day depending on sex and age) to lessen the risk of colon cancer.
  - Eat at least 2.5 cups of a variety of fruits and vegetables daily (linked to lowered incidence of many types of cancer and obesity, which affects the risk for cancer development).
    - Foods high in vitamin A (dark green, red, and orange vegetables)
    - Foods high in vitamin C (citrus fruits)
    - Cruciferous vegetables (broccoli, cauliflower, cabbage)
  - Consume whole grains rather than processed or refined grains and sugars. Low-fiber foods and foods high in fat can cause a variety of cancers (lung, esophageal, pancreatic, oral cavity, cervical, kidney, bladder, liver, stomach).
  - Avoid meat prepared by smoking, pickling, charcoal and grilling, and use of nitrate-containing chemicals (possibly carcinogenic).
  - Consume polyunsaturated and monounsaturated fats (found in fish and olive oil), which might be beneficial in lowering the risk of many types of cancer.
  - Limit alcohol consumption (associated with many types of cancers).
- **Therapeutic nutrition**
  - Cancer can cause anorexia, increased metabolism, and negative nitrogen balance.
  - Systemic effects result in poor food intake, increased nutrient and energy needs, and catabolism of body tissues.
  - An individualized plan is based on the following. Qpcc
    - Increased caloric needs ranging from 25 to 35 cal/kg/day (depending on metabolism, activity level, disease state, and ability to absorb nutrients).
    - Protein needs are increased to 1.0 to 2.5 g/kg/day.
    - Vitamin and mineral supplementation is based upon the client's needs.

HIV/AIDS

The body's response to the inflammatory and immune processes associated with HIV increases nutrient requirements. Malnutrition is common and is one cause of death in clients who have AIDS.

- HIV infection, secondary infection, malignancies, and medication therapies can cause manifestations and adverse effects that impair intake and alter metabolism.
- Decreased nutrient intake occurs due to physical manifestations (anorexia, nausea, vomiting, diarrhea). Psychological manifestations can include depression and dementia.
- Nutritional findings include rapid weight loss, gastrointestinal problems, inadequate intake, increased nutrient needs, food aversions, fad diets, and supplements.
- Poor nutritional status leads to wasting and fever, further increasing susceptibility to secondary infections.
- HIV-associated wasting is characterized by unintended weight loss of 10% and at least one concurrent problem (diarrhea, chronic weakness, or fever) for at least 30 days.
- Diarrhea and malabsorption are prominent concerns in clients who have AIDS.
- Lipodystrophy can cause insulin resistance, altered glucose tolerance, and hyperlipidemia.

Therapeutic nutrition

- Creating an individualized plan for the client who has HIV/AIDS is based on reducing unintentional weight loss and wasting.
  - Increased caloric needs ranges from 37 to 55 cal/kg.
  - A high-protein diet is recommended with amounts varying from 1.2 to 2.0 g/kg/day.
  - Intake of a multivitamin that meets 100% of the recommended daily servings is sufficient, unless a specific deficiency is identified.
- Enteral feedings are used if the client is unable to consume sufficient nutrients, calories, and fluid.
- Liberal fluid intake is extremely important to prevent dehydration.

CLIENT EDUCATION: Consume small, frequent meals that are composed of high-protein, high-calorie, nutrient-dense foods.

COMPLICATIONS

Early satiety and anorexia

CLIENT EDUCATION

- Eat small amounts of high-protein foods loaded with calories and nutrients.
- Try to consume food in the morning when appetite is best.
- Avoid food odors.
- Do not fill up on low-calorie foods (liquids, broth, high-roughage foods containing water).
- Eat cool or room temperature foods.

Mouth ulcers and stomatitis

CLIENT EDUCATION

- Use a soft toothbrush to clean teeth after eating and at bedtime.
- Avoid mouth washes that contain alcohol.
- Omit acidic, spicy, dry, or coarse foods.
- Include cold or room-temperature foods in the diet.
- Cut food into small bites.
- Try using straws.
- Replace meals with high-calorie/protein drinks.
- Use well-fitting dentures.
- Prepare foods that are cooked until tender and soft.
- Add gravies, broth, and a variety of mild sauces to moistened prepared foods.

Fatigue

CLIENT EDUCATION

- Eat a large, calorie-dense breakfast when energy level is the highest.
- Conserve energy by eating foods that are easy to prepare.
- Use a meal delivery service.

Food aversions

CLIENT EDUCATION: Eat foods that are well-tolerated and liked prior to treatments (chemotherapy, radiation). Qᴘᴄᴄ

Taste alterations and thick saliva

CLIENT EDUCATION

- Try adding foods that are tart (citrus juices).
- Eat small, frequent meals.
- Try using sauces and seasonings for added flavor.
- Use plastic utensils for eating.
- Suck on mints, candy, or chew gum to remove bad taste in mouth.
- Sweeten meat with apple or cranberry sauce.

Nausea, vomiting

CLIENT EDUCATION

- Eat cold or room-temperature foods.
- Try high-carbohydrate, low-fat foods.
- Avoid fried foods.
- Do not eat prior to chemotherapy or radiation.
- Take prescribed antiemetic medication.
- Sit up for 1 hr after a meal.
- Sip on fluids throughout the day. Try ginger ale or ginger tea.

Diarrhea

CLIENT EDUCATION

- Ensure adequate intake of liquids throughout the day to replace losses.
- Avoid foods that can exacerbate diarrhea (foods high in roughage).
- Consume foods high in pectin to increase the bulk of the stool and to lengthen transition time in the colon.
- Limit caffeine, hot or cold drinks, and fatty foods.

Application Exercises

1. A nurse is instructing a client who has cancer about ways to increase protein and calories in foods. What actions should the nurse include?

2. A nurse is planning a community presentation on nutritional guidelines for cancer prevention. Which of the following instructions should the nurse include? (Select all that apply.)
   A. Increase intake of foods high in vitamin A.
   B. Consume cruciferous vegetables.
   C. Increase intake of red meats.
   D. Consume oils high in saturated fat.
   E. Consume whole grains.

3. A nurse is collecting data from a client who has HIV. Which of the following findings are manifestations of HIV-associated muscle wasting?
   A. Weight gain of 10%
   B. Report of constipation
   C. Fever for 30 days
   D. Stomatitis

4. A nurse is teaching a client who is undergoing cancer treatment about interventions to manage stomatitis. Which of the following statements by the client indicates understanding of the teaching?
   A. "I will try chewing larger pieces of food."
   B. "I will avoid toasting my bread."
   C. "I will consume more food in the morning."
   D. "I will add more citrus foods to my diet."

5. A nurse is planning to teach a client who is receiving treatment for cancer. Match the potential complication with the nursing instructions.

   A. Anorexia   1. Increase fiber intake.
   B. Stomatitis   2. Sit upright after eating.
   C. Diarrhea   3. Consume high protein foods in the morning.
   D. Constipation
   E. Altered taste   4. Use plastic utensils to eat.
   F. Nausea   5. Eat high-pectin foods.
                        6. Brush teeth with a soft toothbrush.

Active Learning Scenario

A nurse in an oncology clinic is reviewing dietary management with a group of clients who have cancer and are undergoing treatment. What instructions should the nurse include in this discussion? Use the ATI Active Learning Template: System Disorder to complete this item.

CLIENT EDUCATION

- Describe three effects of cancer on nutrition.
- Describe three nutritional needs.
- Describe three activities that promote improved nutrition.

Active Learning Scenario Key

Using the ATI Active Learning Template: System Disorder

CLIENT EDUCATION

Effects of cancer on nutrition
- Causes anorexia
- Increases metabolism
- Causes negative nitrogen balance

Nutritional needs
- Increased calories (25 to 35 cal/kg)
- Increased protein (1 to 2.5 g/kg)
- Vitamin and mineral supplementation

Activities
- Eat more on days when feeling better.
- Consume nutritional supplements that are high in protein and/or calories between meals and/or use as meal replacement.
- Substitute whole milk for water in recipes.
- Add milk, cheese, yogurt, or ice cream to foods when cooking.
- Add peanut butter and yogurt as a spread/topping on fruits.
- Coat meats in eggs, milk, and bread crumbs before cooking.
- Treat cancer-associated complications (early satiety, anorexia, mouth ulcers, stomatitis, fatigue, food aversions, altered taste, thick saliva, nausea, vomiting, diarrhea).

Ⓝ *NCLEX® Connection: Physiological Adaptation, Illness Management*

Application Exercises Key

1. When taking actions, the nurse should instruct the client to substitute whole milk for water in recipes, add milk, cheese, yogurt, or ice cream to dishes, use peanut butter as a spread for fruit or crackers, use yogurt as a topping for fruit, and dip meats in eggs, milk, and breadcrumbs before cooking, to increase protein and calories.

Ⓝ *NCLEX® Connection: Basic Care and Comfort, Nutrition and Oral Hydration*

2. A, B, E. **CORRECT:** When generating solutions, the nurse should include in the presentation for clients to increase their intake of foods high in vitamins A and C, eat a diet high in cruciferous vegetables, and consume whole grains to reduce the risk of cancer.

Ⓝ *NCLEX® Connection: Basic Care and Comfort, Nutrition and Oral Hydration*

3. C. **CORRECT:** When recognizing cues, the nurse should identify manifestations of HIV-associated muscle wasting include unintended weight loss of 10%, and at least one concurrent problem, such as diarrhea, chronic weakness, or fever, for at least 30 days.

Ⓝ *NCLEX® Connection: Physiological Adaptation, Alterations in Body Systems*

4. B. **CORRECT:** When evaluating outcomes, the nurse should determine the client understands the teaching when the client states they will avoid toasting bread. Dry, coarse foods such as toast can worsen the manifestations of stomatitis.

Ⓝ *NCLEX® Connection: Basic Care and Comfort, Nutrition and Oral Hydration*

5. A: 3, B: 6, C: 5, D: 1, E: 4, F: 2

When generating solutions, the nurse should plan to instruct the client who has anorexia to consume high protein foods in the morning, when appetite is best. If the client has stomatitis, the nurse should advise them to brush teeth with a soft toothbrush to reduce irritation. The nurse should plan to instruct the client who has diarrhea to eat high-pectin foods to slow movement of stool. The nurse should plan to instruct the client who has constipation to increase fiber intake to decrease peristalsis. If the client has altered taste, using plastic utensils to eat might reduce the metallic taste of foods. If the client has nausea, sitting upright after eating might promote peristalsis and reduce nausea.

Ⓝ *NCLEX® Connection: Basic Care and Comfort, Nutrition and Oral Hydration*

References

Academy of Nutrition and Dietetics. (2021). *Do's and don'ts for baby's first foods.* https://www.eatright.org/food/nutrition/eating-as-a-family/dos-and-donts-for-babys-first-foods

American Academy of Pediatrics (2022). *Breastfeeding recommendations.* http://www.cdc.gov/breastfeeding/recommendations/index.htm

American Academy of Pediatrics. (2022). *Policy statement: Breastfeeding and the use of human milk.* https://doi.org/10.1542/peds.2022-057988

American Academy of Pediatrics. (2022). *Starting solid foods.* https://www.healthychildren.org/English/ages-stages/baby/feeding-nutrition/Pages/Starting-Solid-Foods.aspx

ATI Nursing. (2022). *Engage community health* (1st ed.).

ATI Nursing. (2022). *Engage fundamentals* (1st ed.).

Berman, A., Snyder, S. & Frandsen, G. (2021). *Kozier & Erb's Fundamentals of nursing: Concepts, process, and practice* (11th ed.) e-book. Pearson.

Burchum, J. R. & Rosenthal, L. D. (2022). *Lehne's pharmacology for nursing care* (11th ed.). Elsevier.

Centers for Disease Control and Prevention. (2021, August 24). *When, what, and how to introduce solid foods.* https://www.cdc.gov/nutrition/infantandtoddlernutrition/foods-and-drinks/when-to-introduce-solid-foods.html

Centers for Disease Control and Prevention. (2022). *Frequently asked questions: What are the benefits of breastfeeding?* https://www.cdc.gov/breastfeeding/faq/index.htm#howlong

Centers for Disease Control and Prevention. (March 10, 2021). *About social determinants of health (SDOH).* https://www.cdc.gov/socialdeterminants/about.html

Cherry, B., & Jacob, S. R. (2019). *Contemporary nursing: Issues, trends, & management* (8th ed.). Elsevier.

DeWit, S. C., Stromberg, H. K., & Dallred, C. V. (2021). *Medical-Surgical nursing: Concepts and practice* (4th ed.). Elsevier.

Dudek, S. G. (2022). *Nutrition essentials for nursing practice* (9th ed.). Lippincott, Williams & Wolter.

Duryea, T. K., & Fleischer, D. M. (2022, March 17). *Patient education: Starting solid foods during infancy (Beyond the Basics).* UpTodate. https://www.uptodate.com/contents/starting-solid-foods-during-infancy-beyond-the-basics-

Grodner, M., Escott-Stump, S., & Dorner, S. (2020). *Nutritional foundations and clinical applications: A nursing approach.* (7th ed.). Elsevier.

Halter, M.J. (2022). *Varcarolis' foundations of psychiatric mental health nursing: A clinical approach* (9th ed.). Elsevier.

Hinkle, J. L., Cheever, K. H., & Overbaugh, K. J. (2022). *Brunner & Suddarth's textbook of medical-surgical nursing* (15th ed.). Wolters Kluwer.

Hockenberry, M. J., Wilson, D. & Rodgers, C. (2019). *Wong's nursing care of infants and children* (11th ed.). Elsevier.

Ignatavicius, D. D., Workman, M. L., Rebar, C. R. & Heimgartner, N. M. (2021). *Medical-surgical nursing: Concepts for interprofessional collaborative care.* (10th ed.). Elsevier.

International Dysphagia Diet Standardization Initiative. (2022). *The IDDSI framework.* https://iddsi.org/framework

National Institutes of Health: National Institute on Drug Abuse (March 2018). *Prescription CNS depressants drugfacts.* https://nida.nih.gov/download/22002/prescription-cns-depressants-drugfacts.pdf

Pagana, K. D., Pagana, T. J., & Pagana, T. N. (2022). *Mosby's manual of diagnostic and laboratory tests* (7th ed.). Elsevier.

Potter, P. A., Perry, A. G., Stockert, P. A. & Hall, A. M. (2021). *Fundamentals of nursing* (10th ed.). Elsevier.

Stanhope, M. & Lancaster, J. (2020). *Public health nursing: Population-centered health care in the community* (10th ed.). Elsevier.

Touhy, T. A. & Jett, K. (2020). *Ebersole & Hess' Toward healthy aging: Human needs and nursing response* (10th Ed.). Elsevier.

U.S. Department of Agriculture. (2020-2025). *MyPlate graphics.* https://www.myplate.gov/resources/graphics/myplate-graphics

U.S. Department of Agriculture. (March, 2018). *Refrigerator & freezer storage chart.* https://www.fda.gov/media/74435/download

U.S. Department of Health and Human Services. (2018). *Physical activity guidelines for americans* (2nd ed.). https://health.gov/sites/default/files/2019-09/Physical_Activity_Guidelines_2nd_edition.pdf

U.S. Department of Health and Human Services. (n.d). *Dietary guidelines for americans.* https://www.dietaryguidelines.gov/sites/default/files/2021-03/Dietary_Guidelines_for_Americans-2020-2025.pdf

U.S. Department of Health and Human Services. (n.d). *Healthy people 2030: nutrition and healthy eating.* https://health.gov/healthypeople/objectives-and-data/browse-objectives/nutrition-and-healthy-eating

U.S. Department of Health and Human Services. (n.d). *Healthy people 2030: overweight and obesity.* https://health.gov/healthypeople/objectives-and-data/browse-objectives/overweight-and-obesity

U.S. Department of Health and Human Services. (n.d). *Healthy people 2030: social determinants of health.* https://health.gov/healthypeople/objectives-and-data/social-determinants-health

U.S. Food & Drug Administration. (n.d.). *Are you storing food safely?* https://www.fda.gov/consumers/consumer-updates/are-you-storing-food-safely

U.S. Food & Drug Administration. (n.d.). *Cold food storage chart.* https://www.foodsafety.gov/food-safety-charts/cold-food-storage-charts

U.S. Food & Drug Administration. (November, 2019). *Nutrition facts.* https://www.fda.gov/media/132225/download

World Health Organization. (2022). *Breastfeeding.* https://www.who.int/health-topics/breastfeeding#tab=tab_2

STUDENT NAME _____

CONCEPT_____ REVIEW MODULE CHAPTER_____

Related Content

(E.G., DELEGATION, LEVELS OF PREVENTION, ADVANCE DIRECTIVES)

Underlying Principles

Nursing Interventions

WHO? WHEN? WHY? HOW?

STUDENT NAME _____

PROCEDURE NAME _____ REVIEW MODULE CHAPTER _____

Description of Procedure

Indications

Interpretation of Findings

CONSIDERATIONS

Nursing Interventions (pre, intra, post)

Client Education

Potential Complications

Nursing Interventions

STUDENT NAME _____

DEVELOPMENTAL STAGE _____ REVIEW MODULE CHAPTER_____

EXPECTED GROWTH AND DEVELOPMENT

Physical Development	Cognitive Development	Psychosocial Development	Age-Appropriate Activities

Health Promotion

Immunizations	Health Screening	Nutrition	Injury Prevention

STUDENT NAME _____

MEDICATION _____ REVIEW MODULE CHAPTER_____

CATEGORY CLASS_____

PURPOSE OF MEDICATION

Expected Pharmacological Action

Therapeutic Use

Complications

Medication Administration

Contraindications/Precautions

Nursing Interventions

Interactions

Client Education

Evaluation of Medication Effectiveness

STUDENT NAME _____

SKILL NAME_____ REVIEW MODULE CHAPTER_____

Description of Skill

Indications

CONSIDERATIONS

Nursing Interventions (pre, intra, post)

Outcomes/Evaluation

Client Education

Potential Complications

Nursing Interventions

STUDENT NAME _____

DISORDER/DISEASE PROCESS _____ REVIEW MODULE CHAPTER_____

Alterations in Health (Diagnosis)

Pathophysiology Related to Client Problem

Health Promotion and Disease Prevention

ASSESSMENT

Risk Factors

Expected Findings

Laboratory Tests

Diagnostic Procedures

SAFETY CONSIDERATIONS

PATIENT-CENTERED CARE

Nursing Care

Medications

Client Education

Therapeutic Procedures

Interprofessional Care

Complications

STUDENT NAME _____

PROCEDURE NAME _____   REVIEW MODULE CHAPTER_____

Description of Procedure

Indications

Outcomes/Evaluation

CONSIDERATIONS

Nursing Interventions (pre, intra, post)

Client Education

Potential Complications

Nursing Interventions

STUDENT NAME _____

CONCEPT ANALYSIS_____

Defining Characteristics

Antecedents

(WHAT MUST OCCUR/BE IN PLACE FOR
CONCEPT TO EXIST/FUNCTION PROPERLY)

Negative Consequences

(RESULTS FROM IMPAIRED ANTECEDENT —
COMPLETE WITH FACULTY ASSISTANCE)

Related Concepts

(REVIEW LIST OF CONCEPTS AND IDENTIFY, WHICH
CAN BE AFFECTED BY THE STATUS OF THIS CONCEPT
— COMPLETE WITH FACULTY ASSISTANCE)

Exemplars